The Global Threat of New and Reemerging

INFECTIOUS DISEASES

Reconciling U.S. National Security and Public Health Policy

Jennifer Brower • Peter Chalk

Supported by The RAND Corporation

RAND
Science and Technology

This research was conducted by RAND as part of its continuing program of self-sponsored research. RAND acknowledges the support for such research provided by the independent research and development (IR&D) provisions of RAND's contracts for the operation of its Department of Defense federally funded research and development centers.

Library of Congress Cataloging-in-Publication Data

The global threat of new and reemerging infectious diseases : reconciling U.S. national security and public health policy / Jennifer Brower, Peter Chalk.
    p. cm.
    "MR-1602-RC."
    Includes bibliographical references.
    ISBN 0-8330-3293-3
    1. Communicable diseases—Social aspects. 2. National security. 3. Bioterrorism—Health aspects. 4. Emergency medical services—Government policy. 5. Emergency management. I. Brower, Jennifer, 1967– II. Chalk, Peter.

RA643.5 .G564 2003
363.3'2—dc21

2002036756

RAND is a nonprofit institution that helps improve policy and decisionmaking through research and analysis. RAND® is a registered trademark. RAND's publications do not necessarily reflect the opinions or policies of its research sponsors.

Cover design by Stephen Bloodsworth

© Credit: R.D.R./Custom Medical Stock Photo
Description: astrovirus from stool colorized

Published 2003 by RAND
1700 Main Street, P.O. Box 2138, Santa Monica, CA 90407-2138
1200 South Hayes Street, Arlington, VA 22202-5050
201 North Craig Street, Suite 202, Pittsburgh, PA 15213-1516
RAND URL: http://www.rand.org/
To order RAND documents or to obtain additional information, contact Distribution Services: Telephone: (310) 451-7002;
Fax: (310) 451-6915; Email: order@rand.org

With the end of the Cold War, there has been a growing realization that the United States and the international community face a number of transnational challenges that do not emanate directly from the policies of individual states. In turn, these challenges cannot be countered solely by the actions of a state, yet they threaten the most basic element of state security, the individual. One important emerging transnational threat in this regard is the spread of infectious disease. This menace has garnered growing attention and resources from the U.S. government since the attacks of September 11, 2000, and the subsequent anthrax attacks.

This report undertakes to examine the changing nature of security and focuses on the threat of infectious disease. It examines two case studies: HIV/AIDS in South Africa as an example of the pervasive and insidious threat disease can pose to a state's stability and security and the threat of infectious disease in the United States to examine the factors in the increasing threat, America's capacity to respond, and policies, institutions, and procedures that can be developed to mitigate the threat.

This report will be of interest to U.S. and international policymakers inside and outside government and at all levels who are developing strategies to cope with the increasing threat posed by pathogens. It should also be of interest to those individuals developing strategies to cope with the emerging security environment.

This study was conducted by RAND Science and Technology as part of RAND's continuing program of self-sponsored research. We acknowledge the support for such research provided by the independent research and development provisions of RAND's contracts for the operation of its Department of Defense federally funded research and development centers. These include Project AIR FORCE (sponsored by the U.S. Air Force), the Arroyo Center (sponsored by the U.S. Army), and the National Defense Research Institute (sponsored by the Office of the Secretary of Defense, the Joint Staff, the unified commands, and the defense agencies).

Questions about the report should be addressed to Jennifer Brower (brower@rand.org) or Peter Chalk (chalk@rand.org) at RAND, 1200 South Hayes Street, Arlington, Virginia, 22202.

RAND is a nonprofit institution that helps improve policy and decisionmaking through research and analysis. RAND Science and Technology (S&T), one of RAND's research units, assists government and corporate decisionmakers in developing options to address challenges created by scientific innovation, rapid technological change, and world events. RAND S&T's research agenda is diverse. Its main areas of concentration are science and technology aspects of energy supply and use; environmental studies; transportation planning; space and aerospace issues; information infrastructure; biotechnology; and the federal R&D portfolio.

Inquiries regarding RAND Science and Technology may be directed to:

Steve Rattien
Director, RAND Science and Technology
RAND
1200 South Hayes Street
Arlington, VA 22202-5050
703-413-1100 x5219
www.rand.org/scitech

CONTENTS

FIGURE

TABLES

SUMMARY

Today, the United States and most of the world face little danger from direct military assault from an opposing state. This threat has been supplanted with concerns about "gray area" challenges that face the global community. Emerging security threats such as terrorism, drug trafficking, and environmental degradation differ significantly from traditional statecentric paradigms both in their causes and the policies designed to ameliorate them.

The increasing transnational threat of infectious disease deserves special attention within this context of the evolving definition of security in the post–Cold War era. Statecentric models of security are ineffective at coping with issues, such as the spread of diseases that originate within sovereign borders, but have effects that are felt regionally and globally. Human security reflects the new challenges facing society in the 21st century. In this model, the primary object of security is the individual, not the state. As a result, an individual's security depends not only on the integrity of the state but also on the quality of that individual's life.

Infectious disease clearly represents a threat to human security in that it has the potential to affect both the person and his or her ability to pursue life, liberty, and happiness. In addition to threatening the health of an individual, the spread of disease can weaken public confidence in government's ability to respond, have an adverse economic impact, undermine a state's social order, catalyze regional instability, and pose a strategic threat through bioterrorism and/or biowarfare.

While infectious diseases are widely discussed, few treatises have addressed the security implications of emerging and reemerging illnesses. This report provides a more comprehensive analysis than has been done to date, encompassing both disease and security. It comes at a critical juncture, as the magnitude and nature of the threat is growing because of the emergence of new illnesses such as Acquired Immune Deficiency Syndrome (AIDS), Ebola, and hepatitis C; the increasing inability of modern medicine to respond to resistant and emerging pathogens; and the growing threat of bioterrorism and biowarfare. In addition, human actions amplify these trends by putting us in ever-greater contact with deadly microbes. Globalization, modern medical practices, urbanization, climatic change, and changing social and behavioral patterns all serve to increase the chance that individuals will come in contact with diseases, which they may not be able to survive.

The AIDS crisis in South Africa provides a disturbing example of how a pathogen can affect security at all levels, from individual to regional and even to global. Approximately one-quarter of the adult population in South Africa is Human Immunodeficiency Virus (HIV) positive, with the disproportionate burden of illness traditionally falling on the most economically and personally productive segment of society. The true impact of the AIDS epidemic is yet to be felt. Deaths from full-blown AIDS are not projected to peak until the period between 2009 and 2012, and the number of HIV infections is still increasing.

The disease is responsible for undermining social and economic stability, weakening military preparedness, contributing to increases in crime and the lack of a capability to respond to it, and weakening regional stability. Specific effects include creating more than two million orphans, removing about US$22 billion from South Africa's economy, and limiting South Africa's ability to participate in international peacekeeping missions.

Many causes played a role in the development of the crisis, including promiscuous heterosexual sex, the low status of women, prostitution, sexual abuse and violence, a popular attitude that dismisses risk, as well as the failure to acknowledge the magnitude of the problem in the early and middle stages of the epidemic. The South African government has made a relatively small effort to curb the epidemic, in part due to President Thabo Mbeki's public questioning of the link between HIV and AIDS, and this has had devastating results. This example serves as a lesson to other countries; if unaddressed, infectious disease can negatively and overwhelmingly affect a state's functions and security.

Currently the United States is managing the infectious disease threat; however, there are many indications that, if left unchecked, pathogens could present a serious threat to the smooth functioning of the country. Many of the global factors that serve to increase the threat from pathogenic microbes are particularly relevant for the United States. These include globalization, modern medical practices, urbanization, global climatic change, and changing social and behavioral patterns. Deaths from infectious illnesses average approximately 170,000 per year, but the scope of the situation is much larger when stigmatization, productivity losses, and other psychological and economic costs are taken into account. In addition, the ability of pathogens to mutate and to spread into previously unknown habitats means that the toll could increase significantly. In the second half of the 20th century almost 30 new human diseases were identified, and antibiotic and drug resistance grew at an alarming rate. This trend applies equally to animal diseases. As citizens continue to travel, import food and goods globally, engage in promiscuous sex, use illegal intravenous drugs, encroach on new habitats, and utilize donated blood, their chances of coming in contact with new or more virulent organisms increases. The added threat of bioterrorism intensifies the risk of encountering a life-threatening microbe.

As Americans' exposure to emerging and reemerging pathogens has grown, the country's ability to respond to infectious disease has diminished in many areas. In 1992, the Institute of Medicine recognized this and challenged the nation to respond. Until the terrorist strikes of September 11, 2001, and the subsequent anthrax attacks, the U.S. government at the federal, state, and local levels had largely failed to respond. In 2002, the public health and medical infrastructure across the United States remains variable and in many cases inadequate to deal with naturally occurring or man-made outbreaks of infectious disease. This infrastructure is highly diverse and includes hospitals, clinics, public health laboratories, pharmaceutical companies, veterinarians, universities, and research groups working to reduce the harmful impacts of microorganisms. Resources and responsibilities for responding to disease outbreaks lie mainly with the state, and the Centers for Disease Control and Prevention (CDC) acts as the lead federal entity. Potential responses to an outbreak include education and information campaigns, vaccination, vector control, food recall, isolation, and quarantine. First an outbreak must be recognized, however, and clinicians and public health laboratories play a critical role in this endeavor. Because of the global nature of the issue, the United States must also act internationally to prevent and respond to disease.

As a result of the low priority given to public health over the past 30 years—in part because of the belief that technological advances would solve the challenges posed by microbes—healthcare workers lack the education and training needed to recognize and treat emerging and reemerging illnesses. Technologies at public health departments and laboratories have not kept pace with other developments; vaccine research, development, and manufacturing has been reduced and concentrated in a few companies; and personnel shortages have been induced in nursing, epidemiology, and other public health and medical areas. In addition, there is a general lack of coordination and communication among the myriad federal, state, and local officials involved in fighting the disease threat and those in the private sector.

Certainly the terrorist attacks have focused attention on the need for a strong public health infrastructure, and policymakers have begun to make funds available to address some of the fundamental shortcomings inherent in the system. However, this investment must be sustained, and there is considerable work to do in enhancing overall policy coordination, management, and development.

The federal government should consider playing a more concerted role in providing resources and instituting unified standards for the common defense against the microbial threat, while giving state and local authorities the flexibility to implement programs in a manner that will best meet local needs. Increased federal investment is critical to endeavors at all levels of government and in the private sector; it could provide the basis from which to develop a functional, coherent national policy for combating infectious disease.

In light of this, there are several specific actions that could be initiated to address the shortcomings identified in this study:

- Coordination between public health authorities at all levels of government needs to be substantially enhanced and developed in conjunction with the development of mechanisms that allow for greater interaction across state borders and local boundaries.

- The private sector must be integrated into overall public health efforts, particularly in relation to the research, development, and manufacture of vaccines and antibiotics and the development of microbial surveillance technology.

- A large-scale education and information campaign should be undertaken, explaining the need for regular vaccination and highlighting the importance of disease prevention through such practices as protected sex, the responsible administration of antibiotics, and "clean" needle exchanges for drug users.

- Efforts should be made to augment the supply of healthcare workers currently available in the country.

- Hospitals and emergency health facilities need to develop appropriate emergency plans to respond to new diseases and large patient influxes, such as those that might occur in the aftermath of a bioterrorist attack or the introduction of a serious infectious illness such as Ebola through airplane travel. Medical receiving facilities should have the means to provide surge capacity in hospital beds and other vital functional areas and have in place auxiliary communication systems and power networks.

- More resources need to be invested in foreign governments to help them increase the effectiveness of their internal disease prevention efforts. Useful initiatives that could be undertaken include

  — mutual aid agreements for the sharing of biological intelligence, research, diagnostics, personnel, vaccines, antibiotics, medical devices, and treatment/prevention techniques;

  — help with the creation of dedicated regional health surveillance networks;

— assistance to promote sustainable urban development and regeneration schemes; and

— focused response efforts to contend with specific disease-promoting catalysts, such as unprotected sex and the spread of AIDS and other sexually transmitted diseases (STDs) in southern Africa.

Beyond these six health-oriented initiatives, the United States also needs to revisit how it defines security and formulates mechanisms for its provision. Institutional structures that have traditionally focused on narrow statecentric concerns will have to be expanded and developed to accommodate challenges that threaten broader societal interests. Increased cooperation among agencies and departments that have historically had little to do with one another—including defense, justice, intelligence, public health, agriculture, and environment—will also be required, as will new executive functions to coordinate such multidimensional policy responses.

One specific area calling for drastic change is the field of national intelligence. The Intelligence Community as a whole will have to become familiar with new operational contexts that require different analytical techniques, skills, mandates, and information-handling methods. Threat assessments and forecasts will need to be grounded on scientifically formulated models that integrate the work of the medical research sector on new and reemerging diseases. Just as important, security analysts will need to work with public health officials and devote greater attention to the epidemiological literature to track new threats. Overseas monitoring activities will also need to encompass a somewhat wider ambit, focusing on such things as the effectiveness of national medical screening systems; prevailing geopolitical, social, economic, and environmental conditions that affect disease incidence; and state compliance with international health conventions and agreements. Indeed, countries that do not pose an obvious military security danger may be the ones most likely to pose a disease risk owing to poorly developed and underfunded public health systems. Such possibilities will need to be recognized and factored into strategic threat analyses.

Given the influence that the United States retains in such major military/security-focused organizations as the North Atlantic Treaty Organization (NATO), Washington could, finally, play a leading role in adapting these institutions to take on a more specific public and global health role. In developing such mandates, the United States could usefully capitalize on the nascent multitask framework that has already been established to perform collective political, military, and humanitarian missions around the world.

Measures such as these will require active political input and sustained financial commitment. Reform along the lines suggested above will require federal resources as well as a better understanding of public health issues and how they affect national and global resilience and stability. Considerable policy attention and resources are flowing to build defenses against the relatively unlikely scenario of a large-scale bioterrorist attack. Responses to more commonly occurring and currently more taxing natural outbreaks remain relatively overlooked and underfunded. Serious assessments of the threat posed by infectious diseases suggest that this imbalance needs to be addressed, as a matter of both fiscal responsibility and judicious public policy.

The nature of security has changed in the post–Cold War era. It now bears little, if any, similarity to the relatively stable bipolar division of East-West power that defined international politics for most of the 20th century. There is no large and obvious equivalent of the Soviet Union against which to balance the United States, the world's sole remaining superpower. Indeed, few of today's dangers have the character of direct military aggression emanating from a clearly defined sovereign source. Instead, security, conflict, and the definition of general threat have become more diffuse and opaque, lacking the simple dichotomies of the Cold War era.

A common thread running through many of the "gray area" influences facing the global community is their transnational and amorphous character. Threats cross international borders but generally cannot be linked directly to the foreign policies or behavior of other states; in addition, they involve patterns, processes, and effects that typically manifest themselves in an ambiguous and highly unpredictable manner. The perceived need for rapid policy responses, therefore, is often "concealed" by and subordinated to prerogatives that are more concrete and more easily discerned in a political sense.

The transnational spread of disease represents one issue that warrants especially close attention within this evolving context. Although not new—viruses and bacteria are as old as human life itself—the nature and magnitude of the threat posed by infectious pathogens are greater today than they have ever been in the past, developments in modern science notwithstanding. Not only have deadly and previously unimagined illnesses, such as AIDS, Ebola, Creutzfeldt-Jakob disease, and Legionnaires' disease, emerged in recent years, but established diseases that just a few decades were thought to have been tamed are also returning, many in virulent, drug-resistant varieties.

Statecentric paradigms are clearly unable to deal with issues such as the spread of diseases that originate within national borders but transcend international boundaries and affect the security of people worldwide. This report represents an effort to provide a more comprehensive, holistic definition of security by focusing on the multidimensional nature of the threat posed by infectious disease. The study specifically recognizes that this particular gray area issue is one that cannot be territorially bounded and, therefore, needs to be understood and addressed in a larger global context.

In Chapter Two, we explain an evolving conception of security—human security—and make clear that disease affects societal, political, and economic stability at many levels. We argue that security is not solely a reflection of an individual as part of a secure state, but is a condition that necessarily encompasses wider components such as quality of life.

Chapter Three examines the increasing threat of infectious disease, focusing on "artificial" disease force-multipliers, which serve to greatly exacerbate the incidence and spread of infectious microbes. Each of these factors and its interaction with the spread of disease are discussed.

Chapter Four examines the current HIV/AIDS crisis in South Africa as an extreme example of the all-embracing threat posed by infectious disease. We assess the impact of HIV/AIDS on the country's internal human and wider geostrategic stability and follow this with an examination of Pretoria's response to the epidemic. We also consider the relevance of the South African case, both regionally and in relation to the wider international system.

In Chapters Five and Six, our discussion turns to threat and preparedness in the United States. While the average American is free of fear from death by infection, microorganisms still pose a significant and increasing threat to the country. Many of the factors discussed in Chapter Three regarding the general increased microbial threat apply to the United States, and Chapter Five analyzes the various factors influencing the reemergence of disease in detail.

Chapter Six considers America's overall response capability to microbial agents. It first examines the critical components of U.S. disease prevention and mitigation efforts and then assesses the significance of the main gaps that are currently serving to undermine the effectiveness of the country's overall public health system.

Finally, Chapter Seven outlines our recommendations for mitigating the threat of disease both in America and abroad. We discuss several specific and direct measures that could be instituted to provide more unified and consistent standards of microbial protection across the country. In addition, we look at institutional reform in the security field and consider how structures that have traditionally focused on narrow, statecentric concerns can be expanded to accommodate challenges that threaten broader societal interests.

ACKNOWLEDGMENTS

This report and the work it represents were made possible by the generous support of RAND and, particularly, by the leadership of Brent Bradley, Stephen Rattien, and James Thomson.

The authors wish to express their thanks to Michael Stoto of RAND and Paul Smith of the Asia-Pacific Center for Security Studies, both of whom provided highly useful and insightful comments on the draft version of this study. A special debt of appreciation is also owed to Matt Wheeler, whose excellent research assistance at RAND was integral to the timely completion of the report.

The authors have benefited from numerous discussions with representatives from the U.S. government at all levels as well as government and academic representatives in South Africa. We would like to acknowledge specifically the time spent by the following individuals:

- Patty Quinlisk, M.D., M.P.H., Medical Director and State Epidemiologist for the Iowa Department of Health

- Colonel Benedict Diniega, M.D., Program Director, Preventive Medicine and Surveillance, Office of Assistant Secretary of Defense

- Samantha Willan, Health Economics and HIV/AIDS Research Division, University of Natal, South Africa

- Dr. John Porter, Department of Infectious and Tropical Diseases, London, School of Hygiene and Tropical Medicine, United Kingdom

- Lindy Heinecken, Centre for Military Studies, University of Stellenbosch, South Africa

- Dr. Stephen Field, South African National Blood Service, South Africa

- Martin Schönteich, Institute for Security Studies (ISS), Pretoria, South Africa

- Mark Colvin, Medical Research Council (MRC), Durban, South Africa.

Any errors of fact and judgment are those of the authors. The views and recommendations expressed herein are not necessarily those of RAND or any of its sponsors.

ABBREVIATIONS

AFB   Air Force base
AIDS   Acquired Immune Deficiency Syndrome
APHIS   Animal and Plant Health Inspection Service
APHL   Association of Public Health Laboratories
ART   Antiretroviral treatment
ATSDR   Agency for Toxic Substances Disease Registry
BIDS   Border Infectious Disease Surveillance
BSL   Biosafety level
BT   Bioterrorism
BW   Biowarfare
CBIRF   Chemical and Biological Incident Response Force
CB-RRT   Chemical and Biological Rapid Response Team
CDC   Centers for Disease Control and Prevention
CIA   Central Intelligence Agency
CISET   Committee on International Science, Engineering,
            and Technology
CSTE   Council of State and Territorial Epidemiologists
DARPA   Defense Advanced Research Projects Agency
DoD   Department of Defense
EIN   Emerging Infection Network
EIP   Emerging Infection Program

EIS	Epidemic Intelligence Service
ELC	Epidemiology and Laboratory Capacity
ELR	Electronic Laboratory Reporting
EPI-AIDs	Epidemiological Assistance
Epi-X	Epidemic Information Exchange
ESSENCE	Electronic Surveillance System for Early Notification of Community-Based Epidemics
EWORS	Early Warning Outbreak Recognition System
FDA	Food and Drug Administration
FEMA	Federal Emergency Management Agency
FFDCA	Federal Food, Drug, and Cosmetic Act
FoodNet	Foodborne Disease Active Surveillance Network
FRP	Federal Response Plan
FSIS	Food Safety and Inspection Service
GAO	General Accounting Office
GDP	Gross domestic product
GEIS	Global Emerging Infections Surveillance and Response System
HACCP	Hazard Analysis and Critical Control Point
HAN	Health Alert Network
HDOH	Hawaii Department of Health
HHS	(Department of) Health and Human Services
HIV	Human Immunodeficiency Virus
ICEID	International Conference on Emerging Infectious Diseases
IDSA EIN	Infectious Disease Society of America, Emerging Infection Network
INPHO	Information Network for Public Health Officials
IOM	Institute of Medicine
IS/APHIS	International Services/Animal and Plant Health Inspection Service

ISS	Institute for Security Studies
MRC	Medical Research Council (South Africa)
MSM	Men having sex with men
NARMS	National Antimicrobial Resistance Monitoring System
NDMS	National Disaster Medical System
NEDSS	National Electronic Disease Surveillance System
NIAID	National Institute of Allergy and Infectious Diseases
NIC	National Intelligence Council
NIH	National Institutes of Health
NIP	National Immunization Program
NMRT	National Medical Response Team
NNDSS	National Notifiable Disease Surveillance System
NPS	National Pharmaceutical Stockpile
OEP	Office of Emergency Preparedness
PulseNet	National Molecular Subtyping Network for Food-borne Disease Surveillance
RRAT	Rapid Response and Advanced Technology (Laboratory)
SABTS	South African Blood Transfusion Service
SANDF	South African National Defense Forces
STD	Sexually transmitted disease
TB	Tuberculosis
USAID	U.S. Agency for International Development
USAMRIID	U.S. Army Medical Research Institute of Infectious Diseases
USAMRMC	U.S. Army Medical Research and Material Command
USDA	U.S. Department of Agriculture
WHO	World Health Organization
ZAR	Rand (South African unit of currency)

Chapter One

DISEASE AND HUMAN SECURITY

THE CHANGING NATURE OF SECURITY IN THE POST-COLD WAR ERA

With the collapse of the Soviet bloc in Eastern Europe in the late 1980s and early 1990s, it appeared that the world system could be on the threshold of an era of unprecedented peace and stability. Politicians, diplomats, and academics alike began to forecast the imminent establishment of a new world order, increasingly managed by an integrated international system based on the principles of liberal democracy and the free market.[1] As this new world order emerged, so it was assumed that serious threats to international stability and security would decline commensurately.

However, the initial euphoria that was evoked by the end of the Cold War has now been replaced by a growing sense of unease that non-traditional challenges—so-called "gray area phenomena"[2]—may soon come to assume greater prominence. Such concern has been stimulated by the remarkable fluidity that now characterizes international politics, an environment in which it is no longer apparent

---

[1]For a detailed survey of these proposed changes, see the International Monetary Fund, *The World Economic Outlook*, Washington D.C., 1991, especially pp. 26–27.

[2]For a detailed account of the notion of gray area phenomena, see Peter Chalk, *Non-Military Security and Global Order: The Impact of Violence, Chaos and Disorder on International Security*, London: Macmillan, 2000, Chapter One. See also Jim Holden-Rhodes and Peter Lupsha, "Gray Area Phenomena: New Threats and Policy Dilemmas," *Criminal Justice International*, Vol. 9, No. 1, 1993, pp. 11–17, and their "Horsemen of the Apocalypse: Gray Area Phenomena and the New World Disorder," *Low Intensity Conflict and Law Enforcement*, Vol. 2, No. 2, 1993, pp. 212–226.

exactly what can be done to whom and with what means. Moreover, it appears that in this new world order turmoil and chaos are increasingly emanating from undefined sources, while violence itself is largely being used by the "weak," not so much as a means of expressing identity but as a way of creating it.[3] Such dynamics are likely to reduce interstate conflict, but only at the expense of an increase in transnational threats that fall below the level of conventional warfare.[4]

Stated more directly, the geopolitical landscape that now faces the global polity lacks the relative stability of the linear Cold War division between East and West. There is no large and obvious equivalent to the Soviet Union against which to balance the United States, the world's sole remaining superpower. Instead, the definitions of security, conflict, and general threat are more diffuse and opaque, existing in the absence of the simple dichotomies that underscored the Cold War era.[5] In commenting on this new environment, former Central Intelligence Agency (CIA) Director James Woolsey remarked: "We have slain a large dragon, but are now finding ourselves living in a jungle with a bewildering number of poisonous snakes. And in many ways, the dragon was easier to keep track of."[6]

A common thread running through many of the threats currently facing the global community—including the spread of disease, the drug trade, environmental degradation, and terrorism—is their transnational character: They cross international borders but generally cannot be linked directly to the foreign policies or behavior of states.[7] Few of today's dangers have the character of direct military

---

[3]See, for instance, "Terrorism and the Warfare of the Weak," *The Guardian* (UK), October 27, 1993.

[4]Richard Latter, "Terrorism in the 1990s," *Wilton Park Papers*, Vol. 44, 1991, p. 2.

[5]See David Abshire, "US Foreign Policy in the Post Cold War Era: The Need for an Agile Strategy," *Washington Quarterly*, Vol. 19, No. 2, 1996, pp. 42–44, and Simon Dalby, "Security, Intelligence, the National Interest and the Global Environment," *Intelligence and National Security*, Vol. 10, No. 4, 1995, p. 186.

[6]James Woolsey, as quoted in John Ciccarelli, "Preface: Instruments of Darkness—Crime and Australian National Security," in John Ciccarelli, ed., *Transnational Crime: A New Security Threat?* Canberra: Australian Defence Studies Centre, 1996, p. xi.

[7]Richard Matthew and George Shambaugh, "Sex, Drugs and Heavy Metal," *Security Dialogue*, Vol. 29, No. 2, 1998, p. 163.

aggression emanating from a clearly defined sovereign source. Rather, these dangers tend to evolve as "threats without enemies," with sources internal rather than external to the political order that the concept of "national interest" has traditionally represented.[8] Unlike the challenge posed by traditional concerns, such as overt aggression, the threats emanating from contemporary gray area influences are far more ambiguous in their patterns, processes, and effects. In many cases, this obfuscates the perceived need for rapid policy responses. Action is typically initiated only after a major crisis destabilizing stage has been reached within the state(s) concerned.[9]

Making sense of these changes will require a holistic, nonlinear approach to security that goes beyond the relatively parsimonious assumptions of realpolitik that have informed international politics for so many years. Traditional spatial notions of security, of national stability defined purely in terms of territorial sovereignty and integrity—which is reflected on a larger scale by the containment policies of the Cold War—simply do not work in today's more complex geostrategic environment. Such statecentric paradigms are clearly unable to deal with issues that originate within national borders but whose effects transcend international boundaries and affect the security of people worldwide.[10] The concept of human security recognizes that individual security is not solely a reflection of an individual as part of a secure state, but also encompasses consideration of quality of life. As Matthew and Shambaugh observe, "[T]oday we must . . . broaden our perspective to encompass neglected areas in which new threats are intensifying, vulnerabilities are real, and forward looking policies are required."[11]

---

[8]Abshire, "US Foreign Policy in the Post Cold War Era," pp. 42–44; Dalby, "Security, Intelligence, the National Interest and the Global Environment," p. 186.

[9]Chalk, *Non-Military Security and Global Order*, p. 3; Holden-Rhodes and Lupsha, "Gray Area Phenomena," p. 12; and William Tow "Linkages Between Traditional Security and Human Security," in William Tow, Ramesh Thakur, and In-Taek Hyun, eds., *Asia's Emerging Regional Order: Reconciling Traditional and Human Security*, Tokyo: United Nations University Press, 2000, pp. 13–21.

[10]Chalk, *Non-Military Security and Global Order*, p. 2. See also Dalby, "Security, Intelligence, the National Interest and the Global Environment," p. 186, and Alan Dupont, "Regional Security Concerns into the 21st Century," in Ciccarelli ed., *Transnational Crime: A New Security Threat?*, pp. 72–73.

[11]Matthew and Shambaugh, "Sex, Drugs and Heavy Metal," p. 163. See also Seyom Brown, "World Interests and the Changing Dimensions of World Security," in Michael

THE CONCEPT OF HUMAN SECURITY

Human security has its intellectual roots in the psychological theories of W. E. Blatz. His observations of individual learning processes and how humans interrelate with society and authority led him to conclude that security is necessarily "all inclusive and pervasive" and is something that does not necessarily require "the protective armor of an agent."[12] The concept also draws heavily on the notions of common and comprehensive security, both of which encapsulate the global dimensions of emerging threats and problems and stress the need to achieve security with, rather than against, others.[13]

The core theoretical foundation of human security, however, is derived from the "globalist" school of thought. This particular paradigm asserts that an "international society" has emerged that integrates communications, cultures, and economics in new ways and in a manner that transcends statecentric relations. While globalists point to the many benefits that can flow from the intermingling of cultures and the creation of international societal "norms," they also acknowledge the complexity of such processes and the wide range of new problems related to security and the welfare of humanity that can result. In many cases, these challenges are portrayed as issues that are beyond the capabilities of individual states to control or, indeed, manage.[14]

The key idea behind human security, and its main contribution to the globalist argument, is the focus on the *individual* as the primary

Klare and Daniel Thomas, eds., *World Security: Challenges for a New Century,* New York: St Martin's Press, 1994, pp. 10–26; James Rosenau, *Turbulence in World Politics: A Theory of Change and Continuity,* Princeton, N.J.: Princeton University Press, 1990; and Donald Snow, *National Security: Enduring Problems in a Changing Defense Environment,* New York: St. Martin's Press, 1991.

[12]W. E. Blatz, *Human Security: Some Reflections,* Toronto: University of Toronto Press, 1966, p. 63. See also Tow, "Linkages Between Traditional Security and Human Security," pp. 13–21.

[13]Ramesh Thakur, "From National to Human Security," in Stuart Harris and Andrew Mack, eds., *Asia-Pacific Security: The Economics-Politics Nexus,* Sydney: Allen and Unwin, 1997, pp. 67–68.

[14]Tow, "Linkages Between Traditional Security and Human Security," p. 19, Anthony Giddens, *The Consequences of Modernity: Self and Society in the Late Modern Age,* Stanford, Calif.: Stanford University Press, 1990; Martin Shaw, *Global Society and International Relations,* Cambridge, Mass.: Polity Press, 1994.

object of security.[15] Canadian Foreign Minister Lloyd Axeworthy, perhaps the most conspicuous exponent of the concept, has listed "safety for people from both violent and nonviolent threats" as core preconditions. He has further emphasized that, "[f]rom a foreign policy perspective, human security is best understood as a shift in perspective or orientation. It is an alternative way of seeing the world, taking people as its point of reference, rather than focusing exclusively on the security of territory or governments."[16]

More specifically, human security recognizes that an individual's personal preservation and protection emanate not just from safeguarding the state as a single political unit, but also from ensuring adequate access to welfare and quality of life.[17] As Thakur observes, this has a dual aspect:

> Negatively, it refers to freedom from: want, hunger, attack, torture, imprisonment without a free and fair trial, discrimination on spurious grounds, and so on. Positively, it means freedom to: the capacity and opportunity that allows each human being to enjoy life to the fullest without putting constraints upon others engaged in the same pursuit. Putting the two together, human security refers to the quality of life of the people of a society or polity. Anything which degrades their quality of life—demographic pressures, diminished access to or stock of resources, and so on—is a security threat. Conversely, anything which can upgrade their quality of life—economic growth, improved access to resources, social and political empowerment, and so on, is an enhancement of human security.[18]

---

[15]Tow, "Linkages Between Traditional Security and Human Security," p. 19.

[16]Lloyd Axeworthy, "Human Security: Safety for People in a Changing World," Department of Foreign Affairs and International Trade, Ottawa, April 1999. See also Astri Suhrke, "Human Security and the Interest of States," *Security Dialogue,* Vol. 30, No. 3, 1999, p. 269.

[17]George McLean, "The United Nations and the New Security Agenda," available at http://www.unac.org/canada/security/mclean.html. See also Keith Krause and Michael Williams, "From Strategy to Security: Foundations of Critical Security Studies," in Keith Krause and Michael Williams, eds., *Critical Security Studies,* Minneapolis: University of Minnesota Press, 1997, p. 43.

[18]Thakur, "From National to Human Security," pp. 53–54.

Human security differs from traditional concepts of security in three important ways. First and most important, the main agent of analysis is the individual rather than the state, and the principal goal is ensuring societal or communitarian stability as opposed to safeguarding territorial sovereignty per se (although, of course, the two objectives are not necessarily mutually exclusive). Second, traditional security stresses structured, militarized interstate violence arising from the existence of an anarchic world as the main threat to international order. By contrast, human security places its emphasis on unstructured chaos and turmoil—which can occur as a result of any number of socioeconomic, political, and environmental factors—as the chief challenge to global stability. Finally, whereas traditional security regards states as competitors whose interactions will always be of a zero-sum nature (i.e., one "wins" only at the expense of another), human security stresses the potential for individual/communitarian cooperation that is undertaken to achieve (absolute) gains that will be to the benefit of all.

Although not intended to be comprehensive, Table 1.1 presents a comparative exploration of these various dimensions for traditional and human security.

While important differences exist, there is one crucial similarity between traditional and human security: both stress the need to reduce the vulnerability of the security subject. Although the two theoretical perspectives differ in their precise account of the source and nature of insecurity, each nevertheless emphasizes the need to employ instruments that can be used to foreclose threatening behav-

Table 1.1

Traditional and Human Security: Comparative Aspects

Traditional Security	Human Security
State	Individual/community
National security	Societal security
Structured violence	Unstructured chaos
Competition	Cooperation
Interactions always lead to relative gains	Interactions can lead to absolute gains

ior and influences.[19] As George McLean notes, both traditional and human security thus "seek to guarantee or guard against some deprivation felt by either the [territorial state], the individual or the community."[20]

THE TRANSNATIONAL SPREAD OF INFECTIOUS DISEASE AS A THREAT TO HUMAN SECURITY

The argument that the transnational spread of disease poses a threat to human security rests on the simple proposition that it seriously threatens both the individual and the quality of life that a person is able to attain within a given society, polity or state. Specifically, this occurs in at least six ways. First and most fundamental, disease kills—far surpassing war as a threat to human life. AIDS alone is expected to have killed over 80 million people by the year 2011, while tuberculosis (TB), one of the virus's main opportunistic diseases, accounts for three million deaths every year, including 100,000 children.[21] In general, a staggering 1,500 people die *each hour* from infectious ailments, the vast bulk of which are caused by just six groups of disease: HIV/AIDS, malaria, measles, pneumonia, TB, and dysentery and other gastrointestinal disorders.[22]

Second, if left unchecked, disease can undermine public confidence in the state's general custodian function, in the process eroding a polity's overall governing legitimacy as well as undermining the ability of the state itself to function. When large-scale outbreaks occur, such effects can become particularly acute as the ranks of first responders and medical personnel are decimated, making it doubly difficult for an already stressed government to respond adequately.

During the initial weeks of the anthrax attacks in fall 2001, the lack of coordination at the federal level, especially with regard to communi-

---

[19]Tow, "Linkages Between Traditional and Human Security," p. 2.

[20]George McLean, "The United Nations and the New Security Agenda," p. 2.

[21]Chalk, *Non-Military Security and Global Order*, pp. 96–97; Laurie Garrett, "Gates Urges More Funds for HIV Prevention," *Washington Post*, April 8, 2001, p. A5.

[22]World Health Organization (WHO), "Report on Infectious Diseases: Removing Obstacles to Healthy Development," available at http://www.who.org/infectious-disease-report/pages/textonly.html, pp. 1–2.

cation, led to a loss of confidence by some citizens, especially postal workers in Washington, D.C. Potentially exposed individuals were given conflicting advice on antibiotic treatment and the efficacy of the anthrax vaccine. The general public, largely because of inconsistent information enunciated by government officials, bought Cipro, the antibiotic approved for the treatment of anthrax, in large numbers.

Similarly, in 1996, Japan suffered a severe food poisoning epidemic caused by *Escherichia coli* O157. Over the course of two months, eight people died and thousands of others were sickened. The perceived inability of the Tokyo government to enact an appropriate response generated widespread public criticism, compounding popular dissatisfaction with an administration that was still reeling from the effects of the previous year's Kobe earthquake. As one commentator remarked at the height of the crisis, "The cries against government authorities are growing louder by the day. . . . The impression here [in Japan] is too much talk and not enough action has led to yet another situation that has spun out of control."[23]

Third, disease adversely affects the economic foundation upon which both human and state security depends. The fiscal burden imposed by the HIV/AIDS epidemic provides a case in point. Twenty-five million people are currently HIV-positive in sub-Saharan Africa, costing already impoverished governments billions of dollars in direct economic costs and loss of productivity. Treating HIV-related illnesses in South Africa, the worst-hit country on the continent, is expected to generate annual increases in healthcare costs in excess of US$500 million by 2009 (see Chapter Three).[24] South and Southeast Asia are expected to surpass Africa in terms of infections by the year 2010. If this in fact occurs, demographic upheaval could tax and widely destabilize countries with fragile economies and public health infrastructures. Economies will be greatly affected by the loss of a stable and productive workforce as well as from a reduction of external capital investment, potentially

---

[23]"Japan Declares E. coli Epidemic an Outbreak: Citizens Accuse Government of Slow Response," CNN Interactive World Wide News, August 1, 1996.

[24]"The Cruelest Curse," *The Economist*, February 24, 2001; Barton Gellman, "An Unequal Calculus of Life and Death," *Washington Post*, December 27, 2000, p. A1.

reducing general gross domestic product (GDP) by as much as 20 percent.[25]

Fourth, disease can have a profound, negative impact on a state's social order, functioning, and psyche. In Papua New Guinea, for instance, AIDS has severely distorted the *wantok* system—which formalizes reciprocal responsibilities, ensuring that those who hit hard times will be taken care of by extended family—because of the fear and stigma attached to the disease.[26] The Ebola outbreak that hit the crowded Ugandan district of Gulu in late 2000 caused people to completely withdraw from contact with the outside world, reducing common societal interactions and functions to a bare minimum.[27] Epidemics may also lead to forms of post-traumatic stress. A number of analyses have been undertaken to assess the long-term psychological effects on those who have been continually subjected to poor sanitary conditions and outbreaks of disease. The studies consistently document the extreme emotional stress suffered by these people and the difficulty of integrating them back into "normal society."[28]

Fifth, the spread of infectious diseases can act as a catalyst for regional instability. Epidemics can severely undermine defense-force capabilities (just as they distort civilian worker productivity). By galvanizing mass cross-border population flows and fostering economic problems, they can also help create the type of widespread volatility that can quickly translate into heightened tension both within and between states. This combination of military, demographic, and fiscal effects has already been created by the AIDS crisis in Africa. Indeed, the U.S. State Department increasingly speculates that the disease will emerge as one of the most significant "conflict

---

[25]See National Intelligence Council (NIC), "The Global Infectious Disease Threat and Its Implications for the United States," NIE-99-17D, Washington, D.C., January 2000, p. 10.

[26]M. O'Callaghan, "PNG-Positive," *Australian Magazine [Weekend Australian],* November 13–14, 1999.

[27]"Deadly Ebola Bug Strikes Uganda," *The New Straits Times,* [Malaysia]. October 18, 2000.

[28]Chalk, *Non-Military Security and Global Order,* pp. 113–114; D. W. FitzSimons and A. W. Whiteside, "Conflict, War and Public Health," *Conflict Studies,* Vol. 276, 1994, p. 28.

starters" and possibly even "war outcome determinants" during the next decade.[29]

Finally, disease can assume a highly significant strategic dimension, through the threat of biowarfare (BW) and/or bioterrorism (BT). Considerations of virulence, morbidity, and rapidity of infectious spread would make the threat far greater than that posed by conventional or even chemical weapons.[30] International attention on BW and BT has increased over the last ten years, particularly in the United States, due to a number of factors:

- Anthrax attacks in fall 2001

- Discoveries of the scope of Iraq's BW efforts after the Persian Gulf War

- Revelations by Boris Yeltsin and Ken Alibek[31] about the depth and breadth of the Soviet Union's BW program

- Evidence that Aum Shinrikyo was actively trying to acquire and disseminate biological agents both prior to and after its 1995 sarin nerve gas attack in Tokyo

- Indications that terrorist organizations not sponsored by states, including Osama bin Laden's al-Qaeda network, have an interest in developing a BT capability.[32]

The consequences of a large-scale, successful act of BW or BT would be catastrophic. Whereas the spread of most infectious diseases spread slowly through natural processes of contagion, deliberate, large-scale releases of virus or bacteria, especially in unvaccinated populations, would lead to the immediate exposure of a specific tar-

---

[29]Center for Strategic and International Studies, *Contagion and Conflict: Health as a Global Security Challenge,* Washington, D.C.: 2000, p. 21; U.S. Department of State, "United States Strategy on HIV/AIDS," publication no. 10296 (July 1995), available at http://dosfan.lib.uic.edu/ERC/environment/releases/9507.html, p. 30.

[30]Chalk, *Non-Military Security and Global Order,* p. 111.

[31]Ken Alibek, *Biohazard,* New York: Random House, 1999.

[32]See, for instance, Center for Strategic and International Studies, *Contagion and Conflict,* p. 12; Ron Purver, "Chemical, Biological, Radiological and Nuclear (CBRN) Terrorism," Perspectives Report 2000/02, Ottawa: CSIS, December 18, 1999; and "Bin Laden Goes After Big Guns," NBC Interactive News, June 15, 2000, available at http://www.msnbc.com/news/421013.

get to a large quantity of (possibly enhanced) infectious organisms. The result would be a massive, largely simultaneous outbreak of disease after an incubation period of only a few days. This would not only cause widespread casualties and panic, but also severely strain and possibly collapse entire public health and response capacities.[33]

Although the emergence and reemergence of disease is a widely discussed topic, only a few assessments have considered a discrete security focus that captures the multicausal and reciprocal mosaic outlined above.[34] Most studies focus specifically on the sources and epidemiological etiology of particular viral and bacterial strains,[35]

---

[33]Richard Falkenrath, "Confronting Nuclear, Biological and Chemical Terrorism," *Survival,* Vol. 40, No. 3, 1998, pp. 45–46.

[34]Selected works (excluding surveys that are purely scientific/diagnostic in nature) include George Armelgaos, "The Viral Superhighway," *The Sciences,* Vol. 38, No. 1, 1998; Institute of Medicine, Committee for the Study for the Future of Public Health, Division of Health Care Services, *The Future of Public Health,* Washington, D.C.: National Academy Press, 1988; Ruth Dircks, ed., *Disease and Society: A Resource Book,* Canberra: Australian Academy of Science, 1989; P. Epstein, "Emerging Diseases and Ecosystem Instability: New Threats to Public Health," *American Journal of Public Health,* Vol. 85, 1995; S. Foster and S. Lucas, *Socioeconomic Aspects of HIV and AIDS in Developing Countries: A Review and Annotated Bibliography,* Public Health Policy Departmental Publication No. 3, London: London School of Hygiene and Tropical Medicine, 1991; L. Garrett, *Betrayal of Trust: The Collapse of Global Public Health,* New York: Hyperion Press, 2000; M. Gregg, ed., *The Public Health Consequences of Disasters,* Atlanta: CDC, 1989; John Last, *Public Health and Human Ecology,* Stamford, Conn.: Appleton and Lange, 1998; M. Lechat, "The Epidemiology of Health Effects of Disasters," *Epidemiological Review,* Vol. 12, 1990; James Logue, "Disasters, the Environment and Public Health: Improving Our Response," *The American Journal of Public Health,* Vol. 86, No. 9, 1996; Bernard Roizman, ed., *Infectious Diseases in an Age of Change,* Washington, D.C.: National Academy Press, 1995; Joseph Smith, "The Ellison-Cliffe Lecture: The Threat of New Infectious Diseases," *Journal of the Royal Society of Medicine,* Vol. 86, 1993; Derek Yach, "The Globalization of Public Health I: Threats and Opportunities," *American Journal of Public Health,* Vol. 88, No. 5. 1998; WHO, *Removing Obstacles to Healthy Development: WHO Report on Infectious Diseases,* 1999, available at http://www.who.org/home/reports.html, accessed January 15, 1999; and National Science and Technology Council, *Infectious Disease—A Global Health Threat,* report of the Committee on International Science, Engineering, and Technology, September 1995.

[35]Some rare exceptions include Dennis Pirages, "Microsecurity: Disease Organisms and Human Well-Being," *Washington Quarterly,* Vol. 18, No. 4, 1995; Jack Chow, "Health and International Security," *Washington Quarterly,* Vol. 19, No. 2, 1996; E. Chivian "Microorganisms, Disease and Security, Technology, Social Change, Demography," *Technology Review,* November/December 1994; Laurie Garrett, "The Return of Infectious Disease," *Foreign Affairs,* January/February 1996; FitzSimons and Whiteside, "Conflict, War and Public Health"; and Alan Whiteside and David FitzSimons,

while much of the security-oriented literature tends to emphasize only one facet of the overall microbial threat: the use of bioagents as offensive or terrorist weapons.[36] If the true dimensions of the challenge posed by infectious and pathogenic organisms are to be understood and factored into viable policy responses, it is vital that more comprehensive and inclusive analyses of *both* disease *and* security be adopted. Only then will policymakers appreciate the full extent of the disease threat with which they are currently faced and, just as important, the socioeconomic and political context within which it operates.

"The AIDS Epidemic: Economic, Political and Security Implications," *Conflict Studies*, Vol. 251, 1992.

[36]See, for instance, Ken Alibek, *Biohazard*; Seth Carus, *Bioterrorism and Biocrimes: The Illicit Use of Biological Agents in the 20th Century*, Washington, D.C.: Center for Counterproliferation Research, National Defense University, 1999; Richard Falkenrath, Robert Newman, and Brad Thayer, *America's Achilles' Heel: Nuclear, Biological and Chemical Terrorism and Covert Attack*, Cambridge, Mass: MIT Press, 1998; D. Henderson et al., "Smallpox as a Biological Weapon: Medical and Public Health Management," *JAMA*, Vol. 281, No. 2, 1999; Ron Purver, "Chemical and Biological Terrorism: A New Threat to Public Safety?" *Conflict Studies*, Vol. 295, 1996; Joshua Lederberg, ed., *Biological Weapons: Limiting the Threat*, Cambridge, Mass.: MIT Press, 1999; Ronald Atlas, "Combating the Threat of Biowarfare and Bioterrorism: Defending Against Biological Weapons Is Critical to Global Security," *Bioscience*, Vol. 49, No. 5, 1999; and Al Venter, "Biological Warfare: The Poor Man's Atomic Bomb," *Jane's Intelligence Review*, March 1999.

Chapter Two

FACTORS ASSOCIATED WITH THE INCREASED INCIDENCE AND SPREAD OF INFECTIOUS DISEASES

The bubonic plague that swept across Europe during the Middle Ages, the smallpox that was carried to the Americas by the Spanish, and the influenza outbreak of 1918 all bear testimony to the historic relevance of infectious pathogens and their ability to cause widespread death and suffering. In many ways, however, the nature and magnitude of the threat posed by infectious pathogens are greater today than they have ever been in the past, developments in modern science notwithstanding. Emerging and reemerging infections present daily challenges to existing medical capabilities. Not only have deadly and previously unimagined illnesses, such as AIDS, Ebola, Creutzfeldt-Jakob disease, and Legionnaires' disease, emerged in recent years, but established diseases that just a few decades ago were thought to have been tamed are also returning, many in virulent, drug-resistant varieties.[1] Modern manifestations of TB, for instance, bear little resemblance to the 19th-century strains that haunted Europe. TB treatment now requires a daily drug regimen that often requires health workers to personally monitor patients to ensure that they are complying with necessary procedures.[2]

In many ways, this situation is a result of the natural balance of forces between people and infectious organisms. By one estimate, there are at least 5,000 kinds of viruses and more than 300,000 species of bacteria that challenge human beings, many of which are

---

[1]George Armelagos, "The Viral Superhighway," p. 24.

[2]See, for instance, Mark Earnest and John Sbarbaro, "A Plague Returns," *The Sciences*, Vol. 33, No. 5, September/October 1993, pp. 17–18.

able to replicate and evolve billions of times in one human genera-tion.[3] These disparities clearly work to the advantage of pathogens, enabling the evolution of ever more virulent strains that quickly out-strip the ability of humans to respond to them. Just as important, however, are "artificial" disease force-multipliers, which are serving to greatly exacerbate the incidence and spread of infectious microbes. Foremost among these are globalization, modern medical practices, accelerating urbanization, climatic change resulting from global warming, and changing social and behavioral patterns. Each of these factors and its interaction with the spread of disease are dis-cussed below.

GLOBALIZATION

The present international system is now more globally interdepen-dent than at any other time in history. Today one can physically move from one part of the world to another in the same time (if not more rapidly than) it used to take to journey between cities or coun-ties. Indeed, no part of the planet remains inaccessible to human penetration, with current estimates of the number of people crossing international frontiers on board commercial flights at more than 500 million every year.[4]

Thanks to developments in transportation technology, this move-ment has become progressively more rapid and affordable, meaning that fewer people are restricted to localized business, employment, and leisure activities. At the same time, differentials in labor, pro-duction, and operating costs, as well as comparative advantages in resource allocations, have led to an increasingly vibrant and active global economic system, characterized by the largely unimpeded flow of goods and commodity-related services.[5]

Whether measured on the basis of information flows, the total vol-ume of world trade and commerce, contact between governments, or

---

[3]Armelagos, "The Viral Superhighway," p. 25.

[4]Derek Yach, "The Globalization of Public Health I," p. 737.

[5]Chemical and Biological Arms Control Institute and the CSIS International Security Program, *Contagion and Conflict; Health as a Global Security Challenge*, Washington D.C.: CSIS, January 2000, p. 3.

links between people, the figures all show major increases, especially over the last 20 years.[6] While it is not necessary to spell out these developments in terms of specific statistics—the trends are both clear and well known—the consequences for the spread and emergence of infectious diseases do require some elucidation.

On one level, the global trade in agricultural products has increasingly brought people into contact with exotic and foreign animal diseases that have subsequently "jumped" across the species line to infect humans. Several examples stand out. In September 2000 a major outbreak of Rift Valley fever hit Saudi Arabia, killing several dozen people in a matter of days. The source of the epidemic was eventually traced back to imports of infected sheep from neighboring Yemen.[7] In Europe, the emergence of the nervous system disorder Creutzfeldt-Jakob disease has been linked to the consumption of beef products originally derived from British cattle afflicted with *bovine spongiform encephalopathy,* or "Mad Cow Disease." And in the United States, the outbreak of West Nile virus in 2000 is now believed to have originated at least partly from the importation of chickens into New York.[8]

On a more direct level, the speed of modern air transportation has greatly facilitated the global transmission of disease among humans. Travelers experiencing either fully developed or incubating endemic or emerging diseases from their departure location can rapidly carry microbes into nonendemic areas. In the United Kingdom and the United States, for instance, there have been numerous cases of people living near major metropolitan airports contracting malaria apparently imported aboard jets operating transcontinental routes.[9] Equally as indicative is typhoid fever. Roughly 400 cases of the disease are reported every year in America, 70 percent of which are

---

[6]Chalk, *Non-Military Security and Global Order,* p. 6.

[7]See, for instance, "Fever Kills 200 in Saudi Arabia and Yemen," Reuters, September 24, 2000, and "Sheep Smuggled from Yemen Responsible for Jizan Outbreak," *Arab News,* September 24, 2000.

[8]Comments made during the International Conference on Emerging Infectious Diseases (ICIED), Atlanta, July 16–19, 2000.

[9]Joseph Smith, "The Threat of New Infectious Diseases," *Journal of the Royal Society of Medicine,* Vol. 86, 1993, p. 376; A. Kondrachine and P. Trigg, "Global Overview of Malaria," *Indian Journal of Medical Research,* Vol. 106, 1997, pp. 39–53.

acquired by individuals while traveling overseas.[10]   Outbreaks of Legionnaires' disease have been similarly linked to such dynamics. As Laurie Garrett observes:

> In the age of jet travel, a person incubating a disease such as Ebola can board a plane, travel 12,000 miles, pass unnoticed through customs and immigration, take a domestic carrier to a remote destination, and still not develop symptoms for several days, infecting many other people before his [or her] condition is noticeable.[11]

Compounding the problem is the fact that overcrowded, poorly ventilated, and (sometimes) unsanitary aircraft constitute ideal environments for the transmission of viruses and bacteria, particularly on long flights. Reflecting this, travel health guidelines issued by the World Health Organization (WHO) now specifically refer to the possibility of catching infectious TB in flight as "realistic," especially on flights of more than eight hours. The WHO has recorded several instances in which individuals flying on planes with other TB-infected travelers have been infected with the bacterium that causes the lung infection.[12]

One disease that has certainly reached pandemic proportions at least partly as a result of globalization and the international movement of goods and people is AIDS. Studies in Africa have tracked the progress of the causative HIV agent along trucking routes, with major roads acting as principal corridors of viral spread between urban areas and other proximal settlements. In one study of 68 truck drivers and their assistants, 35 percent were found to be HIV-positive. Further epidemiological research revealed a wide travel history for these individuals, involving seven different countries served by the ports of Mombassa, including Kenya, Uganda, Zaire, Burundi, and Rwanda. Tourism, especially tourism involving sex, has also played a contributing role. There can be little doubt that the global spread of AIDS has been encouraged by the substantial

---

[10]See "Disease Information: Typhoid Fever," available at http://www.cdc.gov/ ncidod/dbmd/diseaseinfo/typhoidfever_g.htm.

[11]Garrett, "The Return of Infectious Disease," p. 69.

[12]Smith, "The Threat of New Infectious Diseases," p. 376; "WHO Cites Air Travel Risk," Associated Press, December 18, 1998.

patronage of the Asian sex markets and by the equally large number of international travelers visiting such countries as Thailand, India, and the Philippines every year.[13]

MODERN MEDICAL PRACTICES

During the 1960s and 1970s, there was a great deal of hope that humankind had tackled some of its worst infectious diseases through medical advances. This sense of confidence culminated in 1978 when the member states of the United Nations (UN) signed the Health for All, 2000, agreement. The accord set out ambitious goals for responding to infectious diseases among other things, predicting that at least some of the world's poorest and least developed states would undergo a fundamental (positive) health transition before the end of the century.[14]

The optimism inherent in the UN declaration rested on the belief that advances in antibiotics, vaccines, and other remedial treatments—together with striking improvements in food preparation and water treatment—had provided the world's polities with a formidable armory that could be brought to bear against microbial agents. Indeed, just the year before, the WHO had announced the effective eradication of the smallpox virus after the last known case of smallpox had been tracked down and cured in Ethiopia.[15]

While scientific progress has certainly helped to mitigate the effects of certain infectious ailments, overuse and misuse of antibiotics—both in humans and in the agricultural produce they consume—has contributed to a process of "pathogenic natural selection," which is helping to generate ever more resilient, resistant, and powerful dis-

---

[13]Thomas Quinn, "The AIDS Epidemic: Demographic Aspects, Population Biology and Virus Evolution," in Richard Krause, ed., *Emerging Infections,* New York: Academic Press, 1998, p. 331; Thomas Quinn, "Population Migration and the Spread of Types I and 2 Human Immunodeficiency Viruses," in Bernard Roizman, ed., *Infectious Diseases in an Age of Change,* Washington, D.C.: National Academy Press, 1995, p. 81; FitzSimons and Whiteside, "Conflict, War and Public Health," p. 24.

[14]Garrett, "The Return of Infectious Disease," pp. 66–67. See also CDC, "Preventing Emerging Infectious Diseases: A Strategy for the 21st Century," Atlanta: CDC, October 1998, p. 3.

[15]Eradication was not certified officially by the WHO until 1980. Ibid., p. 67.

ease strains. Much of this evolution stems from the rapidity with which microbes are able to adapt and replicate plasmid in their DNA and RNA codes, the genetic dynamic of which commands mutation under stress. Individuals who fail to complete prescribed treatment courses further aggravate the problem by allowing a residual, more resistant viral or bacterial base to survive and flourish.[16]

The result has been the systematic emergence of microbial "super genes" that either offer resistance to several families of antibiotics (or dozens of individual drugs) at any one time or confer greater powers of infectivity and virulence.[17] Very much indicative of this was the emergence of a previously unknown and highly potent derivative of the *Staphylococcus aureus* bacteria in the late 1990s. The microbe has proven so resistant that it is able to survive exposure to vanco-mycin—a so-called "silver bullet" drug that is typically used to treat infections when all other recourses fail. It is believed that part of the reason for the emergence of the enhanced *aurea* strain was an overwillingness to prescribe antibiotics for routine illnesses that could have been cured by the natural workings of immune systems.[18]

Unfortunately, multiple antibiotic resistance and/or increased viru-lence and tolerance are developing in some of the most prevalent and lethal diseases of our time. As noted in Chapter One, strains of *Mycobacterium tuberculosis*, the organism that causes TB, that are resistant to more than one medication have already appeared and are becoming increasingly prevalent not just in the developing world but also in "medically advanced" nations such as the United States (see Chapter Three). Highly resilient varieties of cholera, pneumo-

---

[16]Garrett, "The Return of Infectious Disease," p. 67; "The Global Infectious Disease Threat and Its Implications for the United States," *Foreign Affairs*, Vol. 75, No. 1, January/February 1996, p. 23; "Wonder Drugs at Risk," *Washington Post*, April 19, 2001, p. A19.

[17]Garrett, "The Return of Infectious Disease," p. 67. Microbes have appeared, for instance, that can grow on a bar of soap, swim in bleach, ignore exposure to higher temperatures, and survive doses of penicillin logarithmically larger than those effec-tive in 1950.

[18]See, for instance, T. L. Smith et al., "Emergence of Vancomycin Resistance in *Staphylococcus aureus*," *New England Journal of Medicine*, Vol. 340, 1999, pp. 493–501; "Antibiotic Resistant Germ Kills Woman, Hong Kong Officials Say," CNN Interactive World Wide News, February 22, 1999. See also CDC, *Preventing Emerging Infectious Diseases*, p. 1.

nia, malaria, dysentery, and typhoid have also emerged and are now prevalent in varying degrees throughout the Asia-Pacific region, Europe, and Africa (see Table 2.1). Influenza, in particular, has exhibited a remarkable ability to change genetically. The phenomenon, termed "antigenic drift," occurs nearly every year and makes it extremely difficult for the body to mount defenses because antibodies against one type of influenza confer little or no immunity against other types or subtypes.[19] "Antigenic shift," which is a more dramatic genetic change, may leave a large proportion of the world's population without protective immunity, which could result in a pandemic if the genetically evolved influenza is easily transmitted between people.[20] Indeed, the Centers for Disease Control and Prevention (CDC) expects that a new, deadly strain of the virus may strike sometime within the next ten years, quite possibly on the same scale as the 1918 outbreak (which killed 21 million people in a matter of months).[21]

Modern medical science and/or associated practices are helping to heighten human vulnerability to viral and bacterial pathogens in other ways. Invasive treatment procedures are exposing people to hospital-acquired infections, including the *S. aureus* bacterium noted above. This is particularly true in the developing world, where typically only the sickest—and, therefore, the most vulnerable—are hospitalized. The use of contaminated blood to make clotting agents and antibody plasma proteins such as gamma globulin has similarly exposed patients to highly debilitating diseases such as AIDS and

---

[19]NIC, "The Global Infectious Disease Threat and Its Implications for the United States," p. 23.

[20]Thomson American Healthcare Consultants, "Guidelines for Prevention and Control of Pandemic Influenza in Healthcare Institutions," March 23, 2000, available at http://www.ahcpub.com/ahc_root_html/hot/breakingnews/flu03232000.html, accessed March 16, 2002.

[21]Comments made by Scott Lillibridge during the Biological and Chemical Preparedness: The New Challenge for Public Health meeting, Decatur, July 19–20, 2000. See also Armelagos, "The Viral Superhighway," p. 24, and Chow, "Health and International Security," p. 63.

Table 2.1

Examples of Drug-Resistant Infectious Agents and Percentage of Infections
That Are Drug Resistant, by Country or Region

Pathogen	Drug	Country/Region	Percentage of Drug-Resistant Infections
Streptococcus pneumonia	Penicillin	United States	10 to 35
		Asia, Chile, Spain	20
		Hungary	58
Staphylococcus aureus	Methicillin	United States	32
	Multidrug	Japan	60
Mycobacterium tuberculosis	Any Drug	United States	13
	Any Drug	New York City	16
	Any Drug	Eastern Europe	20
Plasmodium falciparum (malaria)	Chloroquine	Kenya	65
	Mefloquine	Ghana	45
		Zimbabwe	59
		Burkino Faso	17
		Thailand	45
Shigella dysenteriae	Multidrug	Burundi, Rwanda	100

SOURCES: U.S. Institute of Medicine, 1997; WHO, 1999. Reproduced in NIC, *The Global Infectious Disease Threat and Its Implications for the United States,* p. 23.

hepatitis C—a problem becoming especially prevalent in China, where there exists a thriving illegal trade in blood.[22]

Just as serious are the nature and direction of contemporary medical research, which is exhibiting an increased predilection toward the wholesale eradication (rather than control) of microbial organisms. Significantly, much of this exploratory work is proceeding in the absence of a definitive understanding of the etiology of diseases and the environmental contexts in which they exist. As Joshua Lederberg, a Nobel prize–winning biologist, points out, this is liable to prove a highly costly (and misplaced) "war of attrition" in that it will probably merely upset the delicate ecological balance between

---

[22]See, for instance, Elisabeth Rosenthal, "In Rural China, a Steep Price for Poverty: Dying of AIDS" *New York Times,* October 28, 2000, p. A1; "Out in the Open," *Newsweek,* December 4, 2000; and Elisabeth Rosenthal, "With Ignorance as the Fuel, AIDS Speeds Across China," *New York Times,* December 30, 2001, p. A1.

microbes and their human hosts and, in so doing, exacerbate overall individual vulnerability to pathogenic infections and mutations.[23]

Further, improved medical practices have extended the lives of many ill people whose immune systems are less capable of combating microorganisms. An increasing number of individuals in the United States and elsewhere are living with HIV/AIDS infection, cancer, transplanted organs, and aged immune systems. The presence of these people raises the likelihood that opportunistic pathogens will take hold.

ACCELERATING URBANIZATION

At the turn of the 20th century, only 5 percent of the globe's inhabitants lived in cities with populations over 100,000. By the mid-1990s, more than 2.5 billion people resided in metropolitan centers.[24] Most of this urban growth has taken place in the poorer parts of the world. In 1950, for instance, roughly 18 percent of the population of developing states lived in cities. By 2000, the number had jumped to 40 percent, and by 2030 it is expected to reach 56 percent. Several of these conglomerations will have populations in excess of ten million inhabitants. Indeed, according to the UN, 24 so-called "megacities" have already surpassed this demographic threshold, including Jakarta, Calcutta, Lagos, Karachi, and Mexico City.[25]

The reasons for the high rate of rural-urban migration throughout the developing world are complex and varied. However, they typically incorporate factors such as drought, flooding, and other natural disasters; an excess of agricultural labor; sociopolitical unrest generated by civil war; a lack of employment opportunities; and rural banditry. Fleeing these types of conditions (or variations of them), millions of dispossessed workers have moved to squalid shantytowns on the outskirts of major third-world cities, swelling urban popula-

---

[23]Comments made by Joshua Lederberg during the ICEID, Atlanta, July 16–19, 2000.

[24] Eugene Linden, "The Exploding Cities of the Developing World," *Foreign Affairs*, Vol. 75, No. 1, January/February 1996, p. 53.

[25]These figures come from the UN's Population Division and are based on 2000 estimates. Data in Eric Pianin, "Around Globe, Cities Have Growing Pains," *Washington Post*, June 11, 2001, p. A9.

tions and overloading already inadequate water, sanitary, medical, food, housing, and other vital infrastructural services. These expanding metropolitan hubs are proving to be excellent breeding grounds for the growth and spread of infectious bioorganisms.[26] According to one study, a lack of clean water, sanitation, and hygiene alone account for an estimated 7 percent of all disease-related deaths that occur globally.[27]

Asia in particular has been severely hit by the negative interaction between unsustainable city growth and disease spread. The region's urban population is currently estimated to be 1.1 billion. By 2025, it is expected to have risen to 3.8 billion and Asia will contain half the world's people—more than half of whom will live in cities. Nine of the aforementioned "megacities" already exist in the region, including Beijing, Calcutta, Jakarta, Mumbai (formerly Bombay), Osaka, Shanghai, Tianjin, and Tokyo.[28]

Many of these cities lack the basic infrastructure funding necessary to provide proper roads, sewers, housing, and sanitation systems— all essential if economic productivity and a minimal standard of living are to be sustained. According to the Asian Development Bank, 13 of the world's 15 most polluted cities are in the Asia-Pacific region, some rivers of which are thought to carry up to three to four times average world levels of fecal pollutants.[29] The infectious consequences of these developments are inevitable, with widespread outbreaks of typhoid, malaria, dengue fever, dysentery, and cholera a common occurrence. As Eugene Linden observes:

> Advances in sanitation and the discovery of antibiotics have given humanity a respite from the ravages of infectious disease. But many

---

[26]Last, *Public Health and Human Ecology*, pp. 347–348; Armelagos, "The Viral Superhighway," p. 28; Garrett, "The Return of Infectious Disease," p. 71.

[27]The results of the *World Resources 1998–1999: A Study on the Global Environment* study were reported in "Polluted Environment Causing Worldwide Illness and Deaths," *Manila Times* (Philippines), May 24, 1998. The study used scientific data to explore the relationship between environment and death and disease around the world.

[28]Figures are from the Asian Development Bank as cited in "Rise of the Megacity," *The Australian*, April 24, 1997. See also "Chinese City Portrays Good and Bad of Rapid Growth," *Bangkok Post*, October 12, 1997.

[29]"Cleaning Up in Asia," *The Australian*, May 19, 1997.

epidemiologists [now] fear that this period is drawing to a close as urban growth outruns the installation of sanitation in the developing world and resilient microbes discover opportunities in the stressed immune systems of the urban poor.[30]

Unsustainable urbanization can affect the spread of disease in other ways. Rapid intrusion into new habitats has disturbed previously untouched life forms and brought humans into contact with pathogens and contaminants for which they have little, if any, tolerance.[31] Mushrooming cities in the developing world are also helping to transform oceans into breeding grounds for microorganisms. Epidemiologists have warned, for instance, that toxic algal blooms, fed by sewage, fertilizers, and other industrial and human contaminants from coastal metropolises in Asia, Africa, and Latin America contain countless viruses and bacteria. Mixed together in what amounts to a dirty "genetic soup," these pathogens can undergo countless changes, mutating into new, highly virulent antibiotic strains that can be quickly diffused by nautical traffic. The devastating cholera epidemic that broke out in Latin America in 1991, for instance, occurred after a ship from Asia unloaded contaminated ballast water into the harbor of Callao, Peru. The epidemic, which originated from a resistant strain of the El Tor serogroup, subsequently spread to neighboring countries, infecting more than 320,000 people and killing 2,600.[32]

ENVIRONMENTAL FACTORS

Over the past century, humanity has dramatically affected the global biosphere in deep and complex ways. One important effect of such actions has been a gradual increase in the earth's average surface temperature, a change that many scientists now believe has the potential to actively contribute to the transnational spread of disease. According to two 2001 UN studies by the Intergovernmental

---

[30]Linden, "The Exploding Cities of the Developing World," p. 56.

[31]Armelagos, "The Viral Superhighway," p. 28. This occurred during the early colonization of the United States as well as in Europe at the height of the Industrial Revolution.

[32]Armelagos, "The Viral Superhighway," p. 28; Linden, "The Exploding Cities of the Developing World," p. 57.

Panel on Climate Change, the earth's temperature could rise between 1.4 and 5.8 degrees Celsius over the 1990 average surface temperature during the next century.[33]

Global warming could expose millions of people for the first time to malaria, sleeping sickness, dengue fever, yellow fever, and other insect-borne illnesses. In the United States, for instance, a slight increase in overall temperature would allow the mosquitoes that carry dengue fever to survive as far north as New York City. Also, the insects that carry the *Plasmodium falciparum* parasite, which causes malaria, thrive in the warm climates of the tropics. Increased temperatures in more temperate areas could, conceivably, provide a habitat suitable for the increased distribution of these anopheline vectors.[34]

Of particular concern are the studies that show an association between climatic events and outbreaks of diseases that have already occurred in several parts of the world. Instances of malaria in Madagascar, India, Ethiopia, and Peru have been attributed to sudden increases in mosquito densities resulting from higher rainfall patterns in arid and semiarid regions.[35] Epidemics of cholera, typhoid, and dengue fever in Venezuela, Peru, and Bangladesh and plague in

---

[33]See C. D. Harvell et al., "Climate Warming and Disease Risks for Terrestrial and Marine Biota," *Science*, June 21, 2002, pp. 2158–2162; L. Cifuentes et al., "Hidden Health Benefits of Greenhouse Gas Mitigation," *Science*, August 17, 2001, Vol. 293, pp. 1257–1259; J. T. Houghton et al., eds., *IPCC Third Assessment Report: Climate Change 2001—The Scientific Basis*; and James McCarthy et al., eds., *IPCC Third Assessment Report: Climate Change 2001—Impacts, Adaptation, and Vulnerability.* Both reports are available on-line at http://www.ipcc.ch/pub/reports.htm. See also Eric Pianin, "U.N. Report Forecasts Crises Brought on by Global Warming," *Washington Post*, February 20, 2001, p. A6; Eric Pianin, "Two Studies Affirm Greenhouse Gases' Effects," *Washington Post*, April 13, 2001, p. A6; and Philip P. Pan, "Scientists Issue Dire Prediction on Warming," *Washington Post*, January 23, 2001, p. A1.

[34]Armelagos, "The Viral Superhighway," p. 28; Smith, "The Threat of New Infectious Diseases," p. 376; "Changing Climate," *The Australian*, July 15, 1996.

[35]See, for instance, NIC, "The Global Infectious Disease Threat and Its Implications for the United States," p. 24; A. Kondrachine, "Mission Report on Malaria Epidemics in Rajasthan," unpublished WHO report, 1996; A. Kondrachine, "Malaria in Peru," unpublished WHO report, 1997; J. Lepers et al., "Transmission and Epidemiology of Newly Transmitted Falciparum Malaria in the Central Highland Plateau of Madagascar," *Annals of Tropical Medicine*, Vol. 85, 1991, pp. 297–304; and A. Teklehaimanot, "Travel Report to Ethiopia," unpublished WHO report, 1991.

India have similarly been linked to major shifts in vector and infectious agent distributions caused by altered weather patterns.[36]

Global warming and climatic change may also influence the spread of disease by potentially increasing the incidence and magnitude of natural disasters such as landslides, storms, hurricanes, and flooding. Just as in war and conflict, these events invariably lead to the destruction/disruption of vital communication, health, and sanitation infrastructure as well as the displacement of people into overcrowded, makeshift shelters and camps. Such consequences are likely to have direct adverse effects on public health, transforming a disaster area into a potential "epidemiological time bomb."[37]

Hurricane Mitch, which struck Honduras, Nicaragua, Guatemala, and El Salvador in 1998, while not a result of climate change, clearly demonstrated that natural disasters can increase the incidence of infectious illnesses in a population. The desolate landscapes left in the wake of the storm quickly degenerated into disease-ridden slums with children swimming in rivers contaminated by putrefying bodies and flood debris and famished survivors eating animals that had fed on rotting flesh. Cholera and other enteric diseases became especially endemic, their spread facilitated by the lack of clean drinking water, appalling sanitary conditions, and overcrowded shelters. Compounding the problems were impassable roads, wrecked bridges, and poor communications, making the provision of aid and essential medical relief supplies virtually impossible. The catastrophe is one of the worst natural disasters to have hit Central America in 200 years.[38]

---

[36]Karen Day, "Malaria: A Global Threat," in Richard Krause, ed., *Emerging Infections,* New York: Academic Press, 1998, p. 485; "Changing Climate," *The Australian;* "Raining Misery: Millions Marooned in Bangladesh," *Sydney Morning Herald,* September 19, 1998; "A Needy Nation Struggles with Disaster," *Sydney Morning Herald,* September 19, 1998.

[37]See, for instance CSIS, *Contagion and Conflict,* p. 21–22; Logue, "Disasters, the Environment, and Public Health," pp. 1207–1210; Gregg, ed., *The Public Health Consequences of Disasters;* Lechat, "The Epidemiology of Health Effects of Disasters," pp. 192–198; A. McMichael, "Global Environmental Change and Human Population Health: A Conceptual and Scientific Challenge for Epidemiology," *International Journal of Epidemiology,* Vol. 22, 1993, pp. 1–8; and Epstein, "Emerging Diseases and Ecosystem Instability," pp. 168–172.

[38]"Disease Threatens Survivors," *The Australian,* November 9, 1998; "They Survived Mitch—To Live in Misery," *Sunday Times* (Singapore), November 15, 1998.

CHANGES IN SOCIAL AND BEHAVIORAL PATTERNS

Changes in human social and behavioral patterns have had a profound impact on the spread of infectious illnesses. HIV/AIDS represents a case in point. Although the precise ancestry of HIV is uncertain, early transmission of the disease was undoubtedly facilitated by greater acceptance of multiple sexual partners and permissive homosexuality, particularly in nations such as the United States. Today, almost 1.4 million people are living with HIV throughout North America and Western Europe, with some cities, such as New York, among the places in the world where the disease is most prevalent.[39] While the rate of new infections in the developed world slowed during the 1990s (especially in the United States)—largely because of the initiation of effective sex education campaigns and the availability of effective antiretroviral drugs[40]—the disease continues to decimate Africa and South/Southeast Asia (see Table 2.2). Sub-Saharan Africa has been particularly badly affected, where a staggering 21.8 million people have died since the disease was first diagnosed in the early 1980s. Overall, the subcontinent accounts for roughly 70 percent of the world's AIDS cases and three-quarters of its AIDS-related deaths.[41]

In Thailand, Cambodia, and India, thriving sex industries have served to compound already serious problems stemming from greater sexual promiscuity. More than 100,000 cases of AIDS were reported in Thailand between 1994 and 1998. Although an intensive campaign initiated by the government has helped to slow the overall rate of new infections in major centers such as Bangkok, the disease remains a serious problem in northern cities such as Chiang Rai, where roughly 40 percent of female prostitutes are thought to be HIV

---

[39]Whiteside and FitzSimons, "The AIDS Epidemic," p. 7; "Young Bear the Brunt as AIDS Spreads Through the World on a Biblical Scale," *The Independent*, November 25, 1998; Garrett, "The Return of Infectious Disease," p. 72.

[40]It should be noted that the increased availability of effective antiretroviral drugs has, to a certain extent, negatively affected unprotected sex awareness, particularly among young women and men, who are once again beginning to engage in potentially risky behavior (such as engaging in sex with multiple partners).

[41]See "The Spectre Stalking the Sub-Sahara," *The Economist*, December 2, 2000, and Bill Brubaker, "The Limits of $100 Million," *Washington Post*, December 29, 2000, p. A1.

Table 2.2

Regional HIV/AIDS Statistics and Features, End of 2001

Region	Adults and Children Living with HIV/AIDS	Adults and Children Newly Infected with HIV	HIV/AIDS Adult Prevalence Rate (15–49 Years of Age) (Percentage)
Sub-Saharan Africa	28.1 million	3.4 million	8.4
South/Southeast Asia	6.1 million	800,000	0.6
Eastern Europe/Central Asia	1.0 million	250,000	0.5
Latin America	1.4 million	130,000	0.5
East Asia/Pacific	1.0 million	270,000	0.1
North Africa/Middle East	440,000	80,000	0.2
Caribbean	420,000	60,000	2.2
North America	940,000	45,000	0.6
Western Europe	560,000	30,000	0.3
Australia and New Zealand	15,000	500	0.1
Total	40 million	5.0 million	1.2

SOURCE: UNAIDS, "AIDS Epidemic Update—December 2001," available at http://www.unaids.org/publications/index.html.

positive.[42] In Cambodia, nearly half of *all* the country's sex workers are known to be infected by HIV, which causes AIDS. Based on current trends, a staggering 10 percent of the country's population could be infected by 2010.[43] Figures for India are equally as serious. In Mumbai alone, 75 percent of the city's 60,000 to 70,000 prostitutes have contracted the disease, up from just 1 percent in 1990.[44] In total, roughly 3.5 million people are currently thought to be living with the disease in India, a rate of infection that owes much to com-

---

[42]Kenrad Nelson, "Thailand's HIV-Prevention Program Has Slowed the Epidemic, but AIDS-Related Opportunistic Infections Have Increased," Johns Hopkins School of Public Health, May 31, 2001, available at http://www.jhsph.edu/pubaffairs/press/thailands_HIV.html. See also "More Thai Patients Progress to Full-Blown Disease," *Bangkok Post*, March 22, 2001, and "Thai Army Winning AIDS Battle," *Far Eastern Economic Review*, May 5, 1998.

[43]UNAIDS, "AIDS Hits Asia Hard," December 1997, available at http://www.thalidomide.org/FfdN/Asien/asia.html.

[44]UNAIDS, "Aids Hits Asia Hard"; UNAIDS, *HIV/AIDS: The Global Epidemic*, Geneva: UNAIDS Publication, December 1996; UNAIDS, *The Status and Trends of the Global HIV/AIDS Pandemic*, Geneva: UNAIDS Publication, July 1996.

mercial sex and the high levels of sexually transmitted diseases (STDs) in the country.[45]

The increasing prevalence of intravenous drug use has also been instrumental in encouraging the spread HIV/AIDS. Burma, for example, which sits at the heart of the infamous opium-producing "Golden Triangle"[46] and was free of HIV only a few years ago, now has an estimated 200,000 people carrying the virus, 74 percent of whom are intravenous drug users.[47] Equally indicative is India, where intravenous drug use is now the second most common method of transmission for the disease (behind heterosexual sex), something that is especially true in the northeast regions that border Burma.[48] China has been especially hard hit. The Beijing government freely admits that the outbreak of an AIDS epidemic in the country's south is directly related to drug addicts sharing needles to inject heroin. Indeed Ruili, a border town in the southwestern province in Yunnan with one of the highest concentrations of opium addicts in the country, is now in the unenviable position of also being the AIDS capital of China.[49] In Kunming China, 40 percent of intravenous drug users are estimated to be HIV-positive, and because HIV/AIDS education in China is extremely poor, many of these abusers are unknowingly spreading the HIV virus to the general population through sexual encounters and through contaminated blood donations.[50] This resulted in a 67 percent increase between 2000 and 2001 in reported AIDS cases in China.[51]

---

[45]A. Fauci and T. Quinn, "The AIDS Epidemic: Considerations for the 21st Century," *New England Journal of Medicine,* Vol. 341, No. 14, 1999, p. 336; Whiteside and Fitz-Simons, "The AIDS Epidemic," p. 7.

[46]The Golden Triangle is composed of eastern Burma, northern Laos, and northern Thailand. During the 1980s and the first part of the 1990s, the region constituted the world's main source of refined opiates, after which it was superseded by Afghanistan.

[47]Peter Chalk, "Low Intensity Conflict in Southeast Asia," *Conflict Studies,* Vol. 305, No. 306, 1998, p. 12.

[48]World Bank Group, "India's National AIDS Control Program," September 1999, available at http://www.worldbank.org/aids.

[49]Noted in Whiteside and FitzSimons, "The AIDS Epidemic," p. 30.

[50]The vast majority of blood in China is not donated voluntarily. Unsterilized needles, improper practices at blood collection centers, and inadequate laboratory capabilities for blood testing make the blood donation system in China hazardous, although the government has been working to reduce the risk over the past five years. "Keeping China's Blood Supply Free of HIV/AIDS," U.S. Embassy, April 1997, available at

Although HIV/AIDS is the clearest example of how altered social and behavioral patterns have affected the occurrence and spread of infectious disease, it is not the only one. Changes in land use have also played a significant role. The emergence of Lyme disease in North America and Europe has been linked to reforestation and subsequent increases in the deer tick population, while conversion of grasslands to farming in Asia is believed to have encouraged the growth of rodents carrying hemorrhagic fever and other viral infections.[52] In the United States and United Kingdom, the development of large-scale factory farms and increased interactions between rural and urban populations have been linked to outbreaks of *Salmonella* and *cryptosporidiosis* as well as the general increased incidence of zoonotic diseases that are passed from livestock to humans (see Chapter Four).[53]

Finally, as society has moved into habitats requiring environmental modification, niches have been inadvertently created that are proving to be highly conducive for microbial growth and development. Heating and ventilation systems using water cooling processes, for instance, are now known to provide the perfect breeding ground and dissemination pathway for *Legionella pneumophila*, the causative agent of Legionnaires' disease.[54]

Medical science has come a long way in improving our basic understanding of the origin and effect of most infectious diseases humans may contract. Nevertheless, we have proven far less adept at recognizing and effectively dealing with the factors that facilitate the spread of viral and bacterial agents. Through such things as urbanization, climatic change, changing social and behavioral patterns, globalization, and misappropriate/misguided remedial procedures, humanity is rapidly approaching what one commentator has

---

http://www.usembassy-china.org.cn/english/sandt/webaids5.htm, accessed March 13, 2002.

[51]Rosenthal, "With Ignorance as the Fuel, AIDS Spreads Across China."

. [52]NIC, "The Global Infectious Disease Threat and Its Implications for the United States," p. 22.

[53]See, for instance, Lawrence Gostin et al., "Water Quality Laws and Waterborne Diseases: Cryptosporidium and Other Emerging Pathogens," *American Journal of Public Health*, Vol. 90, 2000, pp. 847–853.

[54]Smith, "The Threat of New Infectious Diseases," p. 375.

referred to as the "twilight of the antibiotic era." Not only are we having trouble controlling age-old problems like TB, cholera, and malaria, but new, previously unimagined illnesses and viruses such as HIV/AIDS have emerged with a vengeance.

The impact of HIV/AIDS has been especially devastating and underscores, perhaps more than any other, the pervasive nature of the contemporary microbial challenge. To gain a better understanding of the virus and the disease implications of its spread for wider socioeconomic and political stability, Chapter Three makes a detailed analysis of AIDS in one of the world's most severely affected states, South Africa.

Chapter Three

AIDS IN SOUTH AFRICA: EXTENT, IMPLICATIONS, AND RESPONSE

The contemporary HIV/AIDS crisis in South Africa represents an acute example of how infectious diseases can undermine national resilience and regional stability. Roughly 25 percent of the country's adult population is currently infected with HIV, which makes South Africa one of the most severely affected AIDS states in the world. The consequences of the disease have been as marked as they have been pervasive, negatively impacting on virtually all levels of the country's security—broadly defined—as well as significant aspects of Pretoria's frontline neighbors. As James Wolfenson, president of the World Bank, has remarked:

> Many of us used to think of AIDS as a health issue. We were wrong. AIDS can no longer be confined to the health or social sector portfolios. Across Africa, AIDS is turning back the clock on development. Nothing we have seen is a greater challenge to the peace and stabilities of African societies than the epidemic of AIDS. . . . We face a major development crisis, and more than that a security crisis. For without economic and social hope we will not have peace, and AIDS surely undermines both.[1]

This chapter examines the current AIDS crisis in South Africa and assesses its impact on the country's internal human and wider geo-

---

[1]James Wolfenson, speech given to the UN Security Council meeting on HIV/AIDS in Africa, January 10, 2000, cited in Greg Mills, "AIDS and the South African Military: Timeworn Cliché or Timebomb?" *HIV/AIDS: A Threat to the African Renaissance,* Konrad-Adenauer-Stiftung Occasional Papers, June 2000, p. 67.

strategic stability. We first explain the basic epidemiology of the virus and explore the principal factors associated with its high incidence and spread in South Africa. We then discuss the main security implications of HIV/AIDS, delineating these in terms of human costs, economic development, military preparedness, and civil disorder. We follow this with a critique of Pretoria's response to the epidemic before finally considering the relevance of the South African case, both regionally and to the outside world.

WHAT IS AIDS?

The causative agent of AIDS is HIV, a retrovirus first isolated in 1983 (by Luc Montagnier and Robert Gallo) that works by attacking the CD4 cells, which organize the body's overall immune response to foreign bodies and infections. There are two types of immunodeficiency virus: HIV-1, which has caused most of the infections worldwide, and HIV-2, a more slowly acting mutation of the virus that seems to be concentrated mainly in West Africa.[2] In southern Africa, the dominant strain is HIV-1 (henceforth referred to simply as HIV), at least nine different clades[3] of which have so far been identified.[4]

AIDS normally develops after a median time period of between eight and ten years when an infected person's immune system has been so weakened that it can no longer fight off opportunistic infections, such as pneumonia, TB, and diarrhea, that it would normally be able to resist. TB, in fact, is the most likely cause of death of HIV-positive individuals; in sub-Saharan Africa, for instance, cocontaminations

---

[2]Programme for the surveillance of HIV/AIDS and other sexually transmitted infections (http://www.who.int/emc/diseases/hiv/hiv-surveillance.pdf,) p. 1; Alan Whiteside and Clem Sunter, *AIDS: The Challenge for South Africa,* Cape Town: Human and Rousseau Tafelberg, 2000, pp. 2, 7. For a detailed account of the science around the AIDS virus, see Christopher Wills, *Plagues: Their Origin, History and Future,* London: Flamingo Books, 1997.

[3]*Clade* is a biological term designating a group of organisms that are evolved from a common ancestor.

[4]Author interview, Medical Research Council (MRC), Durban, August 16, 2001. See also Whiteside and Sunter, *AIDS,* p. 2.

occur in more than 80 percent of people afflicted with one or the other of the diseases.[5]

While HIV has proven extremely difficult to fight once a person is infected, it is extremely vulnerable outside the body. The virus must therefore be transmitted through the exchange of bodily fluids, as occurs during such practices as sexual intercourse, blood transfusions, and the sharing of needles. However, because HIV is so fragile, even these modes of infection tend to be inefficient, normally requiring repeated exposure before full acquisition occurs.[6]

The early symptoms of HIV infection typically include chronic fatigue or weakness, severe and sustained weight loss, extensive and persistent swelling of the lymph glands, diarrhea, and severe deterioration of the central nervous system. Full-blown AIDS is characterized by the onset of viral, bacterial, fungal, or parasitic secondary infections caused by pathogens that the immune system can no longer control. Death is caused not so much from the immunodeficiency virus itself as from the opportunistic infections that are its results.[7]

SCOPE AND SPREAD OF HIV/AIDS IN SOUTH AFRICA

Statistics on HIV prevalence in South Africa are derived from annual surveys of pregnant women attending antenatal clinics in the public sector, conducted by the Department of Health. Although this sentinel sample excludes males and females who are either not pregnant or do not register at public sector facilities, it is thought to provide a reasonably accurate assessment of trends occurring among mainstream, sexually active South Africans. Extrapolations to the general population are generally based on two main assumptions: first, that 80 percent of all pregnant women attend public sector antenatal

---

[5]Author interview, London School of Hygiene and Tropical Medicine, London, August 20, 2001.

[6]Author interview, South African Blood Transfusion Service (SABTS), Johannesburg, August 14, 2001.

[7]Whiteside and FitzSimons, "The AIDS Epidemic," pp. 1–4.

clinics; and second, that the ratio of women who are HIV-positive to men who are HIV-positive remains consistent at 1 to 0.73.[8]

In absolute numbers, South Africa has the highest number of HIV-positive citizens of any state in sub-Saharan Africa, which is, itself, the part of the world most severely affected by the epidemic.[9] The most definitive data on the national scope of the virus comes from the Medical Research Council (MRC) in Durban. According to its 2001 report (which was released in fall 2001, despite government attempts to suppress it), 4.7 million South Africans were living with HIV/AIDS as of the end of 2000. This equates to slightly less than 25 percent of the country's total *adult* population (24.5 percent of women attending antenatal clinics in October 2000 tested positive), up from just 0.76 percent in 1990. When children and infants are included, one in nine South Africans is currently thought to be HIV-positive. Of those, 420,000 had developed full-blown AIDS by the

---

[8]Mark Colvin and Eleanor Gouws, "Thukela Water Project Feasibility Study: An Assessment of HIV/AIDS—Its Context and Implications for the TWP," paper provided to the author, August 2001. It should be noted that several commentators in South Africa question the validity of using antenatal surveys to determine the country's overall HIV prevalence. Apart from underrepresenting the middle class and substantial proportions of race groups other than black Africans (through omission of the private sector), biostatisticians also criticize the lack of a consisting sampling frame for the surveys. Above all, they point to the different collection and testing methodologies adopted between the country's provinces, stressing that no centralized control exists over which clinics submit samples or how individual patients are tested (author interviews, MRC, Durban, and SABTS, Johannesburg, August 2001).

[9]According to the WHO, 23 million people were HIV positive in sub-Saharan Africa by the end of 1999, nearly 70 percent of the world's total at that time. Comparative figures for other regions were

- South and Southeast Asia: 6 million
- Latin America: 1.3 million
- North America: 920,000
- East Asia and the Pacific: 530,000
- Western Europe: 520,000
- Caribbean: 360,000
- Eastern Europe and Central Asia: 360,000
- North Africa and the Middle East: 220,000
- Australia and New Zealand: 12,000.

WHO (2000), cited in ING Barings, *Economic Impact of AIDS in South Africa: A Dark Cloud on the Horizon,* London: ING Barings, April 2000, p. 4.

end of 1997.[10] More alarmingly, the MRC report shows AIDS as the leading killer in South Africa, linking no less than 33 percent of all fatalities in the country to the disease. The council projected that by 2002 the virus would account for twice the number of lives lost as a result of either car accidents or murders.[11]

Significant regional variations occur in the republic's HIV incidence levels. The most severely affected province is KwaZulu-Natal, where 36.2 percent of the population is infected with the virus. The Mpumalanga, Gauteng, and Free State administrative districts follow, each with incident rates between 27 and 29 percent. The least affected provinces are the Northern and Western Cape, where prevalence levels currently run at approximately 11 and 8 percent, respectively (see Table 3.1).[12]

The prevalence of HIV/AIDS in KwaZulu-Natal, Mpumalanga, Gauteng, Free State, and North West, relative to the Cape provinces, largely appears to reflect the major transportation routes that connect the country's northern neighbors with cities such as Pretoria, Johannesburg, and Durban. Many of these so-called "frontline states" are severely affected by HIV, the spread of which has been availed by truck drivers who frequently engage in multiple, unprotected sexual encounters (see below).[13] Analysts at the MRC in Durban also believe that the higher incidence rates along the eastern South African corridor are indicative of a higher black-to-white demographic ratio, more acute poverty, and less proactive local government response to AIDS.[14]

---

[10]Department of Health, National HIV and Syphilis Sero-Prevalence Survey of Women Attending Public Antenatal Clinics in South Africa, 2000, available at http://www.doh.gov.za/docs/reports/2000/hivreport.html, p. 6; UNAIDS/WHO Working Group on Global HIV/AIDS and STD Surveillance, "Epidemiological Fact Sheet on HIV/AIDS and Sexually Transmitted Diseases—South Africa," available at http://www.who.ch/emc/diseases/hiv, p. 3.

[11]MRC, *The Impact of HIV/AIDS on Adult Mortality in South Africa*, available at http://www.mrc.ac.za.

[12]Department of Health, National HIV and Syphilis Sero-Prevalence Survey of Women Attending Public Antenatal Clinics in South Africa, p. 7.

[13]Author interview, Institute of Security Studies (ISS), Pretoria, August 13, 2001.

[14]Author interview, MRC, Durban, August 16, 2001.

Table 3.1

Provincial HIV Prevalence Estimates: Antenatal
Clinic Attendees, 1998–2000

Province	Estimated HIV Prevalence Rates (Percentage)		
	1998	1999	2000
KwaZulu-Natal	32.5	32.5	36.2
Mpumalanga	30.0	27.3	29.7
Gauteng	22.5	23.9	29.4
Free State	22.8	27.9	27.9
North West	21.3	23.0	22.9
Eastern Cape	15.9	18.0	20.2
Northern Province	11.5	11.4	13.2
Northern Cape	9.9	10.1	11.2
Western Cape	5.2	7.1	8.7
National	22.8	22.4	24.5

SOURCE: South African Department of Health.

NOTE: True values are estimated to fall within a confidence interval of 95 percent. This should be taken into account when interpreting the data.

As might be expected, the rate of infection is greatest among the 20–29 age group, which tends to be the most sexually active. Statistics for 2000 show an overall prevalence level in this category of nearly 60 percent, compared with 16 percent for the under-20 age group, 24 percent for the 30–34 age group, 16 percent for the 35–39 age group, and between 11 and 13 percent for the 40–49 age group.[15]

South Africa is still far from feeling the full effects of its HIV crisis and, indeed, is really only just emerging from the first phase of the epidemic. Over the next decade, the republic is expected to see further increases in HIV infections—the rates of which are not expected to level off until 2010—accompanied by a rapid surge in AIDS deaths—the incidence of which is projected to peak somewhere between 2009 and 2012 (see Table 3.2).[16] As Martin Schönteich, a

---

[15]Department of Health, National HIV and Syphilis Sero prevalence Survey, p. 8. See also Whiteside and Sunter, *AIDS*, p. 51.

[16]Author interviews, ISS, Pretoria, August 13, 2001; MRC, Durban, August 16, 2001; and University of Cape Town, August 17, 2001.

Table 3.2

Projected AIDS Deaths and AIDS Deaths as a Ratio of
Non–AIDS Related Deaths, 1999–2015

Year	AIDS Deaths per 100 People	AIDS Deaths per 100 Non–AIDS Related Deaths
1999	0.42	57.6
2000	0.56	76.7
2001	0.71	99.2
2002	0.89	124.6
2003	1.07	151.7
2004	1.26	178.7
2005	1.43	203.5
2006	1.57	224.3
2007	1.67	239.9
2008	1.74	249.9
2009	1.78	254.8
2010	1.78	255.5
2011	1.77	253.4
2012	1.74	249.3
2013	1.71	244.4
2014	1.67	239.2
2015	1.64	234.2

SOURCE: Actuarial Society of South Africa.

senior researcher at the Pretoria-based Institute of Security Studies (ISS), remarks, "Most areas of South Africa have only recently begun to move from the asymptomatic HIV phase of the epidemic to the AIDS phase. In simple terms, the people who are visibly ill today are the under one percent who were infected in 1990."[17]

In an attempt to provide greater clarity to the future dynamics of HIV in South Africa, several models have been developed to map the likely progression of the disease over the next 10 to 15 years. One notable project, which was undertaken by Metropolitan Life on behalf of the UN Development Program in 1998, forecasts an overall HIV prevalence rate in 2010 of 6,195,000 infected individuals, with

[17]Martin Schönteich, "Age and AIDS: A Lethal Mix for South Africa's Crime Rate," *HIV/AIDS: A Threat to the African Renaissance?* Konrad-Adenauer-Stiftung Occasional Papers, June 2000, p. 61.

AIDS cases exceeding 800,000.[18] The Actuarial Society of South Africa, working in conjunction with the University of Cape Town, has developed similar mathematical models and predicts that HIV prevalence levels will peak in 2006 at around 16.7 percent of the population as a whole—although certain regions such as KwaZulu Natal are expected to register highs approaching 40 percent.[19]

MAIN FACTORS ASSOCIATED WITH THE SPREAD OF HIV/AIDS IN SOUTH AFRICA

Various factors have contributed to the contemporary HIV/AIDS crisis in South Africa, including heterosexual sex, the low status of women, prostitution, sexual abuse and violence, and prevalent risk-prone attitudes. Each of these causal influences is discussed below.

Heterosexual Sex

In the black population, heterosexual sex remains the main transmission mode for HIV in South Africa. Although drug use is common, unlike in many developed countries, in South Africa most narcotics are either swallowed or smoked; viral infection via the sharing of dirty needles has, as a result, been relatively uncommon.[20] Equally, standards and facilities operated by the South African National Blood Service are world class and equivalent to those in Europe and North America. All blood that is donated for transfusion purposes is vigorously tested and categorized according to a four-fold risk schema, which ensures that only samples with an HIV infection potential of 0.06 percent or less are used.[21] Finally, while unpro-

---

[18]Whiteside and Sunter, *AIDS*, p. 69.

[19]Author interview, University of Cape Town, August 17, 2001. See also ING Barings, *Economic Impact of AIDS in South Africa*, pp. 1, 6.

[20]Author interview, ISS, Pretoria, August 13, 2001. During surveillance of four sentinel sites in Cape Town, Durban, Port Elizabeth, and Gauteng (Johannesburg/Pretoria) carried out in 1998, heroin abuse accounted for only 2 percent of visits to treatment services and only half of these involved injection of the drug. Alcohol was by far the most abused substance, with smoked cannabis and Mandrax accounting for almost all of the remaining cases. See Charles Parry, *South African Community Epidemiology Network on Drug Use, January–June 1998 (Phase 4)*, available at http://www.mrc.ac.za.

[21]Author interview, SABTS, Johannesburg, August 14, 2001.

tected male-to-male sex—now officially known as "men having sex with men" (MSM)—did contribute to the original development of HIV in South Africa's white population, access to well-equipped health clinics combined with increasing awareness about the dangers inherent in traumatic intercourse have helped to mitigate prevalence levels in this particular segment of the population.[22]

Among black South Africans, however, casual, unsafe, and abusive sex remains endemic and has provided a ready-made vector for the spread of HIV—the exchange of bodily fluids. Cultural norms play a substantial role, particularly the general acceptance of multiple partners and preference for unprotected sex wherein the use of condoms is specifically eschewed. Often intercourse is also "dry," involving the use of powders and herbs designed to prevent vaginal lubrication. Such practices obviously lead to increased friction and greatly elevate the risk of viral transmission through internal cuts and lesions.[23]

Low Status of Women

Further exacerbating the situation is the patriarchy inherent in black South African society. Women are commonly regarded as inferior and akin to property, and expectations are for sex to be given whenever and however demanded. Such a duty, entrenched in years of tribal tradition, remains an integral feature of many rural communities and is one that is rarely, if ever, questioned. This ingrained gender structure has negatively affected the empowerment of women and, in so doing, undermined female options for refusing intercourse and/or insisting on safe practices such as the use of condoms.[24]

---

[22]Author interview, MRC, Durban, August 16, 2001.

[23]Author interview, MRC, Durban, August 16, 2001. Similar sentiments were expressed during interviews conducted at the ISS, Pretoria, August 13 2001 and the SABTS, Johannesburg, August 14, 2001. Solomon Benatar, "South Africa's Transition in a Globalizing World: HIV/AIDS as a Window and Mirror," *International Affairs*, Vol. 77, No. 2, 2001, p. 360.

[24]Author interview, ISS, Pretoria, August 13, 2001. See also Anne Blommer et al., "Women's Issues in South Africa," available at http://www.evergreen.edu/users6/menste01/gender.html, and UNAIDS/WHO, "Epidemiological Fact Sheet on HIV/AIDS and Sexually Transmitted Diseases: 2000 Update."

Prostitution

The sex trade has also emerged as a major vector for the spread of HIV in South Africa. Prostitutes are used widely throughout the country, something that is particularly true of long-distance truck drivers and rural-urban migrant mine workers—both of whom are forced to spend long periods of time away from their homes and families.[25] Viral infection rates among these segments of the population have skyrocketed in recent years, both on account of the inherent dangers of multiple partners and the African preference for unprotected sex (commercial truck drivers are known to pay double for intercourse without a condom).[26] During the next three to four years, the prevalence of HIV in the transportation and migrant-concentrated mining (as well as construction) sectors is expected to soar to at least 23 percent, and possibly as high as 29 percent, with prostitution use remaining one of the primary causes of transmission.[27]

---

[25]Apartheid established both migration and prostitution as a way of life for many South Africans. The Bantustan system crammed much of the country's black population into crowded, impoverished homelands, which led to the breakdown of traditional cultural structures. Adults, mainly men, were forced to migrate to large cities to find work, often living for extended periods of time in single-sex hostels that were legally "off limits" to their families (at the system's peak in 1985, 1,833,636 South Africans were working as migrants). Urban prostitution, as a result, became the norm for many male workers, including those married to rural wives. Although there are now fewer migrant workers in the country (South Africans live where they choose), the legacy of apartheid remains: Sectors such as the mining industry continue to rely heavily on a migrant labor force and still provide hostel accommodation for their employees. Moreover, although migration has declined internally within South Africa, it remains a significant source of employment for tens of thousands of individuals living in neighboring states. In 1998, for instance, the South African mining industry employed a total of 198,653 foreign migrants, the bulk of whom came from Lesotho, Botswana, Swaziland, and Mozambique. (See Whiteside and Sunter, *AIDS*, p. 63.)

[26]Author interview, MRC, Durban, August 16, 2001. See also Whiteside and Sunter, *AIDS*, pp. 62–64; Robert Shell, "Halfway to the Holocaust: The Economic, Demographic and Social Implications of the AIDS Pandemic to the Year 2010 in the Southern African Region," in *HIV/AIDS: A Threat to the African Renaissance?* Konrad-Adenauer-Stiftung Occasional Papers, June 2000, Pp 14; and "The Spectre Stalking the Sub-Sahara," *The Economist*.

[27]ING Barings, *Economic Impact of AIDS in South Africa*, pp. 25–26.

Sexual Abuse and Violence

Added to these various factors is a culture of sexual abuse and violence, which is now entrenched in southern Africa and is, in many ways, a product of the lack of female empowerment noted above. Rape has become increasingly common, especially among teenage boys who suffer little, if any, social stigmatization from engaging in the practice. Indeed, in many rural schools, "jock rolling" (gang rape) is regarded as "cool" and generally associated with the most popular and socially confident members of the local community. There has also been a major increase in sexual victimization on account of urban legends and myths.[28] One of the most alarming such myths is the widespread belief that an HIV-infected male can cure his disease by having sex with a virgin. Forced sex between older men and young girls has, as a result, become increasingly common, especially in the viral endemic belts of KwaZulu Natal and Mpumalanga provinces.[29] Overall, roughly 50,000 women are raped every year in South Africa—three times the figure for the United States.[30]

Prevalent Risk-Prone Attitudes

Finally, many black South Africans are simply willing to accept the dangers associated with unsafe sexual practices, such as the frequent use of prostitutes. For most, the predilection toward risk-enhancing behavior stems from a fatalistic attitude borne of past racial abuses suffered under the apartheid system, combined with the extraordinarily high level of internal violence and conflict that the country has experienced over the past five years (Johannesburg currently has one of the highest murder rates of any city outside a war zone).[31]

---

[28]Many of these urban legends stem from illiteracy and a general lack of education. Roughly 60 percent of adults in South Africa are unable to read, most of whom are women living in rural areas.

[29]This particular myth was stressed universally to the author during several interviews conducted with South African health experts, August 13–18, 2001.

[30]Blommer et al., "Women's Issues in South Africa." It has been estimated that enough women are raped every day in South Africa to fill four jumbo jets.

[31]Police statistics project that roughly 220,000 murders will take place in South Africa within the next 10 years. See "S. African Says AIDS Not Biggest Killer," *Washington Post*, August 7, 2001.

Together these have engendered a belief that "life is cheap," an expectation that death may occur at any moment, and a tendency to live for today without valuing tomorrow.[32] As Alan Whiteside observes, this attitude can be summed up in the response: "If AIDS kills me in five years' time, so what?"[33]

Recent statements made by Thabo Mbeki questioning the causal link between HIV and AIDS have also affected attitudes toward sexual practices (see below). The South African President retains considerable influence among the population and his dissenting views on the origins of AIDS—which he attributes to poor living conditions, poverty, malnutrition, stress, and trauma—have undoubtedly helped to mitigate popular concerns about the dangers of engaging in unprotected, multiple-partner sex. Virologists and scientific academics have been especially critical of Mbeki in this regard, charging that the low rate of condom use in South Africa—which in 2000 averaged 21 percent between unmarried partners—can, at least in part, be attributed to the President's widely publicized beliefs.[34]

IMPACT ON SOUTH AFRICA

The impact of HIV/AIDS on South Africa's security and stability has been significant. Not only has the disease led to large-scale human death and suffering, but it has also undermined social and economic stability and weakened military preparedness, and it may yet emerge as one of the most important contributors to crime over the next 10 to 20 years.

The Human Cost

From a purely numerical point of view, HIV/AIDS will have an overwhelming demographic impact on South Africa. More than 500,000

---

[32]Author interview, MRC, Durban, August 16, 2001. Similar sentiments were also expressed during interviews at the ISS, Pretoria, August 13, 2001.

[33]Whiteside and Sunter, *AIDS*, p. 64.

[34]This sentiment was generally expressed to the author during interviews conducted at the MRC, ISS, and SABTS, August 13–16, 2001. See also Whiteside and Sunter, *AIDS*, pp. 4–5, and Health Systems Trust (South Africa), "South African Health Review 2000," available at http://www.hsat.org/za/sahr/2000.

people have already died from the disease, and cumulative numbers are projected to rise to at least six million by 2010.[35] Because most people contract HIV at an early age, the bulk of these fatalities will fall on the young adult population. Premature deaths in the 25–29 age group, for instance, are expected to double over the next eight years because of AIDS, with numbers quadrupling in the 30–39 age category.[36]

Children will also be severely affected. Mortality models estimate that anywhere between 13 and 45 percent of infants born to HIV-infected mothers will contract the disease, either during pregnancy or through breastfeeding.[37] The high figure is especially alarming given that most children who become ill with HIV quickly develop AIDS and almost without exception die within five years of birth. Indeed, infant mortality has already soared from less than 1 percent in 1990 to 24.5 percent in 2000, reversing a positive trend that was frequently upheld as a gauge of Pretoria's overall level of development.[38]

The concentration of HIV/AIDS within these age groups has important ramifications for overall life expectancy in South Africa. This is because high numbers of deaths among children and young adults inevitably means that a large number of life years will be lost. According to statisticians at the University of Cape Town, life expectancy at birth will fall to 40 years by 2010, down from 60 years in 1997.[39] Within the high-risk categories, however, projections are even more dire: For children born with the virus, life expectancy is

---

[35]Author interview, University of Cape Town, August 17, 2001. See also U.S. State Department, "Fact Sheet on South Africa," available at http://www.state.gov/r/pa/bgn/index, and Colvin and Gouws, "Thukela Water Project Feasibility Study: An Assessment of HIV/AIDS—Its Context and Implications for the TWP," p. 6.

[36]Whiteside and Sunter, *AIDS*, p. 75; Shell, "Halfway to the Holocaust," p. 16.

[37]Whiteside and Sunter, *AIDS*, pp. 75–76; Associated Press, "S. Africa Sued for Failing to Distribute AIDS Drug," *Washington Post*, August 22, 2001, p. A14. The South African government consistently refused to provide antiretroviral treatment (ART), a treatment known to prevent transmission of HIV from mother to child, to pregnant women. Recently the Treatment Action Campaign won a legal case that will force the government to provide drugs that could halve the transmission risk.

[38]Author interview, University of Cape Town, August 17, 2001.

[39]Author interview, University of Cape Town, August 17, 2001. See also Whiteside and Sunter, *AIDS*, p. 76, and "The Cruelest Curse," *The Economist*, February 24, 2001.

no more than 2.5 years; for those who contract the disease later in life, between 25 and 30 years. As Robert Shell, director of the Population Research Unit in East London, remarks, "In terms of mortality, it will be as if the South African population of 2010 had been put in a giant time machine and slammed back almost 30 years."[40]

The prevalence of AIDS among young adults is also liable to generate a burgeoning orphan population within South Africa. Nearly one million children under the age of 15 will have lost their mothers to the disease by 2005, a figure that, according to Department of Health estimates, will increase to over two million by 2010.[41] Given the sexually transmitted nature of the disease, it is likely that many of these children will also lose (or already have lost) their fathers, resulting in a dramatic increase in the number of orphans as a percentage of the general population. Not only will these children severely strain the capacity of communities to support them, but they will also be at greater risk of engaging in delinquent and criminal behavior (see "Civil Law and Order and Crime" below).[42]

The various demographic impacts of the HIV/AIDS crisis outlined will be felt most acutely in KwaZulu-Natal province, where most of South Africa's viral infections have occurred. Models developed by Metropolitan Life forecast that AIDS-related deaths in this part of the country will rise from under 60,000 per year in 2000 to in excess of 110,000 by 2010. The practical effect of this near doubling of the mortality rate will be a provincial population that is some 15 percent lower than it would have been in a non-AIDS scenario. Most of these deaths will occur within the 20–39 age group, which will decimate the province's economically productive workforce as well as feed into a growing legion of orphans that is expected to number in excess of 450,000 by 2010—nearly a quarter of the national total.[43]

---

[40]Shell, "Halfway to the Holocaust," p. 16.

[41]A. Kinghorn and M. Steinberg, "HIV/AIDS in South Africa: The Impact and the Priorities," Department of Health document (undated), p. 14, cited in Martin Schönteich, "AIDS and Age: [South Africa's] Crime Time Bomb?" *AIDS Analysis Africa*, Vol. 10, No. 2, 1999, p. 1.

[42]Schönteich, "Age and AIDS: A Lethal Mix for South Africa's Crime Rate," p. 62.

[43]Whiteside and Sunter, *AIDS*, p. 72. See also Colvin and Gouws, "Thukela Water Project Feasibility Study," p. 6.

The Economic Impact

In addition to the huge toll in human lives, HIV/AIDS will significantly affect South Africa's growth and development. Over a quarter
of South Africa's economically active population will have contracted
HIV by 2005, affecting sectors ranging from mining to retail and
insurance. Most infections are expected to occur among semi- and
unskilled workers, but the epidemic will also have a major impact on
the highly trained sectors of the labor force (see Table 3.3). Finance
and business services, for instance, are both forecast to face HIV
prevalence levels between 9 and 11 percent.[44] This will exacerbate
an already serious skills shortage and significantly raise the remu-
neration and replacement costs for high-tech companies.[45]

On a more generic level, the AIDS epidemic will force employers to
adjust their net contributions to worker pension, life, and medical
insurance schemes (the overall premiums for which will be higher

Table 3.3

HIV-Positive Individuals per 100 Workers by Skill
Levels, 1999–2010

Year	Highly Skilled	Skilled	Semi- and Unskilled
1999	10.2	15.5	19.9
2000	11.2	17.5	22.7
2001	12.0	19.1	25.2
2002	12.6	20.5	27.4
2003	12.9	21.5	29.2
2004	13.1	22.2	30.6
2005	13.0	22.6	31.6
2006	12.8	22.8	32.3
2007	12.5	22.7	32.7
2008	12.1	22.5	32.8
2009	11.7	22.1	32.8
2010	11.2	21.7	32.7

SOURCE: Wharton Economic Forecasting, 1999.

---

[44]ING Barings, *Economic Impact of AIDS in South Africa,* pp. 7–8, 25.

[45]"Young, Gifted and Dead," *Sunday Times* (South Africa), July 9, 2000. The cost of
replacing just one skilled laborer has been estimated at ZAR250,000 (approximately
US$31,000).

because of increased demand).[46] For the average company that assumes 66 percent the cost of such benefits, this could add 15 percent to overall wage bills by 2005 and about 30 percent by 2010.[47]

Most firms will attempt to pass on these cost increases to consumers in the form of higher prices. This, combined with the higher premiums for health and medical insurance will result in lower take-home pay and associated household incomes. Domestic savings as a proportion of GDP will, therefore, suffer and are projected to be a full two percentage points lower than they would be in a non-AIDS scenario. In order to support sustained investment demand in the economy, South Africa will need to attract additional foreign inflows to fill the gap. Should this fail to materialize, a domestic savings crunch is liable to ensue, which will drive interest rates higher, further slowing overall GDP growth.[48]

Government expenditures will also be affected by the HIV/AIDS crisis, largely because the medical costs for treating the disease that are not covered by private insurance will have to be borne by the public sector. This will have relevance for most of the unskilled labor force as well as the noneconomically active population. By 2009, it is conservatively estimated that Pretoria will be responsible for around 1,087,000 patients with full-blown AIDS. Assuming treatment costs of ZAR3,750 (US$468.75) per person per year, this will lead to annual increases in healthcare expenditures that over the course of the next eight years will be in excess of ZAR4 billion (US$500 million).[49]

The result of these effects will be strongly negative for South African development. According to ING Barings, GDP growth rates will aver-

---

[46]It has been estimated that demand for private healthcare services and insurance could be at least 11 percent higher by 2010 than it would be in a non-AIDS scenario.

[47]ING Barings, *Economic Impact of AIDS in South Africa*, pp. 11–12; Whiteside and Sunter, *AIDS*, p. 88; Department of Finance, *Budget Review 2000*, Pretoria: Department of Finance, 2000, p. 29.

[48]ING Barings, *Economic Impact of AIDS in South Africa*, pp. 12–14; Whiteside and Sunter, *AIDS*, pp. 88–89.

[49]Data derived from Wharton Economic Forecasting Associates, 1999. See also "Young, Gifted and Dead," *Sunday Times*. This heightened expenditure will exacerbate an already woefully inadequate level of funding for healthcare in general, which currently amounts to less than US$85 per person annually. Obviously, as more people become sick with AIDS, the more this (already) low figure will diminish.

age between 0.3 and 0.4 percent less per year as a result of AIDS, removing some US$22 billion from the economy (see Table 3.4).[50]

The cumulative effect will be heightened poverty, which will undermine the resources that both individuals and the state at large are able to bring to bear to mitigate the effects of HIV/AIDS. This will precipitate a vicious downward cycle, with the disease not only driving underdevelopment, but in so doing, also providing the conditions necessary for its continued spread and proliferation.[51]

The Social Cost

The social implications of the HIV/AIDS crisis are equally profound. Although the full impact of the disease will not be felt for some time,

Table 3.4

The Impact of AIDS on GDP Growth Rates, 2000–2015

Year	Real GDP (Percentage)	Growth (Percentage Point Difference)
2000	0.7	
2001	−1.0	−0.3
2002	−1.2	−0.2
2003	−1.4	−0.2
2004	−1.6	−0.2
2005	−1.9	−0.3
2006–2010	−3.1	−0.4
2011–2015	−4.7	−0.3

SOURCE: Wharton Economic Forecasting, 1999.

---

[50]ING Barings, *Economic Impact of AIDS in South Africa*, p. 30. A similar study—Channing Arndt and Jeffrey Lewis, "The Macro Implications of HIV/AIDS in South Africa: A Preliminary Assessment," The World Bank, August 2000, available at http://www.worldbank.org/afr/wps/wp9.pdf—projects that GDP per capita will be 8 percent less in 2008 than it would be in a non-AIDS scenario, leading to a 17 percent drop in real GDP by 2010.

[51]See, for instance, Alan Whiteside, "HIV/AIDS Implications for Poverty Reduction," *United Nations Development Programme Policy Paper,* 2000, pp. 5–10; Mark Colvin and Brian Sharp, "Communicable Diseases and Poverty in Southern Africa," paper presented at a South African Regional Poverty Network Conference at Human Sciences Research Council, Pretoria, April 26, 2001, pp. 4–5; and Whiteside and Sunter, *AIDS*, pp. 91–92.

there are already indications of the type of problems the country can expect to face. In rural areas, AIDS is reducing the demographic pool from which future community leaders can be drawn and, through debilitation, helping to undermine civil participation in political affairs—both of which bear on the effectiveness of governance in what remains a nascent democratic state.[52]

Just as problematic is the effect that the disease is having on the effort to rebuild the educational system in the postapartheid era. Teacher deaths related to AIDS have risen by more than 40 percent since 2000 and currently stand in excess of 1,011.[53] A severe shortage of both school and university instructors is expected to ensue during the next eight to ten years, which will play havoc with South Africa's residual skills base and overall productive social capital.

On a wider scale, HIV/AIDS is having a profoundly negative psychological influence on victims, their extended families, and the fabric of civil society in which these social "units" exist. The emotional reaction to a positive diagnosis has tended to be far more acute than that to any other fatal illness because of the stigma that surrounds HIV— the disease has frequently led to the ostracization of entire families within their communities—and the fact that patients are usually relatively young when they become infected. Not only have these factors resulted in entrenched feelings of hopelessness, depression, despair, and anger, they have also directly affected the trust, interaction, and cooperation that lie at the heart of any functioning civil society.[54] The long-term effects of these community dynamics will be significant and are liable to continue to impinge on South Africa's human development long after the AIDS epidemic has peaked.

---

[52]Author interview, University of Natal, Durban, August 17, 2001.

[53]Overall numbers of teacher AIDS-related deaths are projected to rise to 12,600 by 2010. See "AIDS Wipes Out [South Africa's] Teachers," *Sunday Times* (South Africa), December 14, 2001; and "AIDS Wipes Out [South Africa's] Teachers," *Sunday Times* (South Africa) (Internet version), available at http://www.Suntimes.co.za/2001/11/94/news/news02.osp, accessed January 10, 2001.

[54]Whiteside and Sunter, *AIDS*, pp. 92–94; Shell, "Halfway to the Holocaust," pp. 19–20.

Military Preparedness

Beyond human, economic, and social considerations is the impact that the current HIV crisis is likely to have on the capabilities and operational effectiveness of the South African National Defense Forces (SANDF). The prevalence of HIV within the military is somewhat difficult to determine due to a lack of publicly available data. However, the SANDF itself has acknowledged that between 10 and 12 percent of its soldiers are infected with the virus. Most commentators within South Africa believe this to be a conservative estimate at best and typically put overall prevalence levels closer to or above the national average of 22 percent. One report in 2000 claimed that as many as 60 to 70 percent of the military could be infected, a figure that is comparable or greater than that of other sub-Saharan armies (see Table 3.5).[55] The bulk of those with HIV are believed to be within the 20–29 age category—the tactical and operational heart of the SANDF—with "guesstimates" of overall prevalence in that category as high as 50 percent.[56]

HIV will undermine the combat readiness, effectiveness, and credibility of the SANDF in a number of ways. As the disease develops, more and more troops will have to be retired from active combat duty and transferred to less demanding support and logistics roles.

---

[55]See "60% of [South African] Army May Be HIV Positive," *Mail and Guardian* (South Africa), March 31, 2000. One unit in the border regions of KwaZulu-Natal has been repeatedly cited as having immunodeficiency rates in excess of 90 percent.

[56]Author interview with representatives from the South African Military Academy, Cape Town, August 18, 2001. See also Mills, "AIDS and the South African Military," p. 70. All those joining the defense forces are required to undergo mandatory HIV testing prior to recruitment and all those identified with the disease are barred from entry. This means that HIV infection within the SANDF occurs after enlistment. There are several reasons accounting for this, notwithstanding the artificially ordered, structured, and isolated nature of the defense forces and the availability of healthcare and counseling services not available to the public at large. Soldiers are predominantly young, sexually active, governed more by peer pressure than established social norms and frequently dislocated from their families. These factors weigh heavily in favor of prostitution use, which, given the self-perceptions of invincibility that troops are typically imbued with, often takes place in the absence of condoms. Exacerbating the situation is the prevailing practice of inoculating combat forces with live attenuated viruses, which, when combined with highly stressful operational environments, is believed to help heighten the overall susceptibility to HIV infection.

Table 3.5

HIV Prevalence Rates in Selected Militaries in
Sub-Saharan Africa

Country	Estimated HIV Prevalence (Percentage)
Angola	40–60
Congo (Brazzaville)	10–25
Cote d'Ivoire	10–20
Democratic Republic of the Congo	40–60
Eritrea	10
Malawi	75
Nigeria	10–20
Tanzania	15–30
Uganda	66
Zimbabwe	80

SOURCE: National Intelligence Council.

This will inevitably lead to a "hollowing out" of the army's operational middle management and a concurrent loss of expertise and experience derived from the SANDF's crucial 20–29 frontline age sector. Moreover, the practical effect of transferring HIV-infected combat personnel to fill backup logistics positions will be the creation of a support component that is both semitrained and increasingly sick.[57]

Development, discipline, and morale are also likely to suffer. Troopers discovering they are HIV-positive will have little incentive to attend training classes (as the possibility for a full military career will be effectively eliminated) and may well be tempted to be increasingly insubordinate (as consequences for disobeying orders will now be measured against the certainty of death). Unit cohesiveness will be similarly affected, both because of disruptions caused by AIDS-related sicknesses and reassignments and because of breakdowns in force collegiality brought about by the general stigmatization of soldiers infected with the virus.[58]

---

[57]Lindy Heinecken, "Strategic Implications of HIV/AIDS in South Africa," *Journal of Conflict and Development*, Vol. 1, No. 1, 2001, pp. 110–112.

[58]Author interview, Cape Town, August 18, 2001. See also Lindy Heinecken, "HIV/AIDS, the Military and the Impact on National and International Security," paper presented at the millennium colloquium of the South African Political Studies Association, Bloemfontein, South Africa, September 20–22, 2000, and Central Intelli-

In addition to causing these organizational problems, AIDS is liable to have a direct bearing on Pretoria's ability to participate in international peacekeeping missions. Current policy is that no HIV-positive personnel should be included in contingents slated for multinational or external duties. In effect, this means that nearly a quarter of the SANDF cannot be deployed overseas, which has greatly impinged on the government's freedom to quickly employ combat units for foreign peacekeeping and peacemaking duties.[59] According to officials with the country's leading military academy, this is one of the main reasons for South Africa's failure to play a more active role in trying to stymie the wave of civil violence that has engulfed the region surrounding the Democratic Republic of the Congo over the past three to four years.[60]

A weakened military will have profound implications for Pretoria, both internally and externally. The nature of civil conflict in South Africa—which combines criminal, political, tribal, religious, and ethnic violence—is well beyond the enforcement capacities of the police, meaning that ultimately mitigation relies on the support of the defense forces. Seen in this light, any decisive reduction in the operational effectiveness of the SANDF is likely to have serious ramifications in terms of South Africa's national security and stability.[61]

Externally, South Africa's inability to play a decisive role in regional peacekeeping missions is liable to undercut the country's credibility as a viable regional hegemon and could act as a source of consider-

---

gence Agency, *Report 2000: The Global Infectious Disease Threat and Its Implications for the United States,* available at http://www.cia.gov/cia/publications/nie/report/nie99-17d.html, pp. 6, 33.

[59]Heinecken, "Strategic Implications of HIV/AIDS in South Africa," p. 111.

[60]Author interview, Cape Town, August 18, 2001. See also Mills, "AIDS and the South African Military" p. 70. Besides these problems, AIDS is also likely to negatively affect the South African defense budget. As more and more soldiers become debilitated with HIV, so too will related healthcare, treatment, and personnel replacement costs rise. In certain sub-Saharan African armies, AIDS victims are already taking up 80 percent of military hospital beds. Replacing these soldiers and ensuring that they have access to sufficient medical resources will require substantial and ongoing investments, which a developing state such as South Africa (not to mention regional South African Development Community neighbors) can ill afford, much less sustain, for the next 10 to 15 years that the epidemic will take to run its course. For further details, see Heinecken, "Strategic Implications of HIV/AIDS in South Africa," pp. 109–110.

[61]Author interview, Cape Town, August 18, 2001.

able political embarrassment—particularly if forces cannot be sent to help contain sudden and widely publicized humanitarian emergencies.[62] Moreover, because Pretoria's military remains the best equipped and trained in sub-Saharan Africa, its absence from regional peacekeeping missions will significantly detract from the effectiveness of any future multinational deployments that are required. Consequently, zones of increased dissidence and conflict could quickly emerge, to the general detriment of stability in South Africa's immediate neighborhood.

Civil Law and Order and Crime

Finally, HIV/AIDS could quite possibly emerge as one of the most important drivers of crime and civil instability in South Africa over the next two decades. One area that security analysts are paying particularly close attention to is the epidemic's likely effect on the number of orphans as a percentage of the country's general population. As previously noted, statistical models project that more than two million South Africans under the age of 15 will have lost their parents to AIDS by 2010 (see Figure 3.1).[63]

Most of these youths will suffer from social and educational isolation as a result of the stigma that is attached to AIDS. Many will also be severely impoverished, particularly given that the loss of income-earning heads of households will occur in what are already the most marginalized and underdeveloped parts of rural South Africa. These two factors are liable to significantly exacerbate the effects of an age-crime correlation, which repeated criminological studies have shown to be at its height during the teenage years, especially when the individual in question lacks parental guidance, role models, and viable economic opportunities.[64] There is, in other words, a danger of AIDS

---

[62]This latter issue would be especially acute if less militarily prepared states were able to respond to regional humanitarian emergencies and make highly visible contributions.

[63]Schönteich, "Age and AIDS: A Lethal Mix for South Africa's Crime Rate," pp. 61–62.

[64]See, for instance, J. Graham and B. Bowling, *Young People and Crime*, Home Office Research Study No. 145, London: Her Majesty's Stationery Office, 1995; T. Newburn, "Youth, Crime and Justice," in M. Maguire, R. Morgan, and R. Reiner, eds., *The Oxford Handbook of Criminology*, Oxford: Clarendon Press, 1997; Home Office Research and

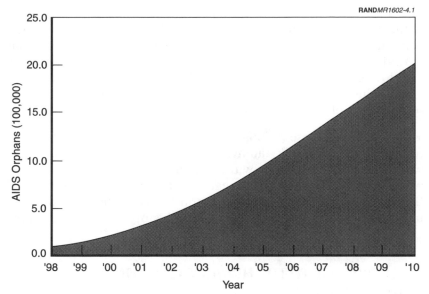

SOURCE: South African Department of Health, Kinghorn and Steinberg, *HIV/AIDS in South Africa: The Impact and Priorities*, undated, p. 1.

Figure 3.1—Number of AIDS Orphans, 1998–2010

helping to produce a juvenile population that is at greater than average risk of engaging in delinquent behavior and exhibiting antisocial tendencies.[65]

Beyond the impact on orphans, the HIV/AIDS epidemic has the potential to negatively affect virtually all aspects of Pretoria's criminal justice system. Not only is the disease projected to have a devastating effect on the effectiveness of the national police—which, given the age and marital structure of the force, is acutely prone to STDs—it is also liable to seriously degrade the efficiency of the judicial legal

Statistics Department, "Information on the Criminal Justice System in England and Wales," London: Her Majesty's Stationery Office, 1995; and Federal Bureau of Investigation, *Crime in the United States, 1996,* Washington D.C.: Department of Justice, 1996.

[65]Martin Schönteich, "The Impact of HIV/AIDS on South Africa's Internal Security," paper delivered at the First Annual Conference of the South African Association of Public Administration and Management, Pretoria, November 23, 2000. See also his "Age and AIDS: A Lethal Mix for South Africa's Crime Rate," pp. 61–63.

system by debilitating and/or killing key players, such as defense witnesses and trial prosecutors. Overall, this will both heighten the general perception that crime pays as well as serve to reduce popular confidence in the institutional enforcement capacity of the state. The former will provide added individual incentives to engage in crime, while the latter will work to exacerbate what is already a serious problem of mob justice and vigilantism.[66]

The net effect of these various developments will be entirely negative for South Africa's civil stability, possibly reducing the country to widespread social anarchy within the next five to 20 years. In the words of one commentator, "As early as 2010, the year in which AIDS [is projected] to equal six million, South African society could be living out the values of a movie gangland dystopia such as [that portrayed in the movie] 'Mad Max.'"[67]

THE RESPONSE TO THE HIV/AIDS CRISIS IN SOUTH AFRICA

The Government Response

Despite the far-reaching and insidious impact that HIV/AIDS is having on South Africa, remarkably little concerted action has been taken by the government to address the disease. Although the true nature of the disease was largely unknown for many years and despite the challenges surrounding Pretoria's own emergence from apartheid to democratic rule, it is generally accepted that far more could have been done and, more to the point, could be done now to stem the crisis.

A significant factor that has hindered government action over the last few years is the attitude of Thabo Mbeki.[68] At the World AIDS Con-

---

[66]Author interview, ISS, Pretoria, August 13, 2001.

[67]Shell, "Halfway to the Holocaust," pp. 18–19.

[68]Other factors have also affected the government's will to take decisive action, including a general lack of health capacity and an entrenched system of patriarchy that has negatively affected the status of women, particularly in the public policy realm. However, most commentators agree that with a different President in place, there would be far greater possibility for South Africa to institute initiatives that could make a meaningful difference in the fight against AIDS. There is some empirical sup-

ference in his own country, the South African President publicly questioned the link between HIV and AIDS, basing his views on the unconventional theories of Peter Duesberg and David Rasnick. Both of these scientists claim that AIDS is neither a new nor an unknown disease maintaining, rather, that it is a collection of preexisting viruses—the potency of which has been exacerbated by the twin effects of poverty and misapplied (Western-developed) pharmaceutical treatments. They also cite cases in which those confirmed with HIV have not developed AIDS as well as a handful of instances in which people have been diagnosed with immunodeficiency similar to AIDS but HIV has not been present to back up their contention that there is no necessary link between the two conditions.[69]

Although Mbeki has now withdrawn from the public debate over the root cause and epidemiology of AIDS, he has not retracted his previous endorsement of Duesberg and Rasnick. There is no doubt that the President's prevailing attitude has served to delegitimize prevention programs that could have been instituted to contain and manage the disease, particularly the use of ARTs. These multidrug programs have been proven to substantially enhance the quality and length of life of HIV-infected persons and now form one of the most important weapons for battling AIDS throughout much of the Western world.[70] These drugs are especially efficient at preventing mother-to-child transmission.

Initially, the high cost of ARTs—which runs to roughly US$10,000 per patient per year in the United States—precluded their use in most developing countries.[71] However, over the past year, international pharmaceutical companies have substantially lowered the price of many of the drugs integral to these treatments to the extent that even the poorest countries in sub-Saharan Africa and the Asia-Pacific

port for this, as can be witnessed in Botswana and Uganda, where proactive government stances are making a difference.

[69]Whiteside and Sunter, *AIDS*, pp. 3–4; *South African Health Review, 2000,* available at http://www.hst.org.za/sahr/2000.

[70]Author interviews, SABTS, Johannesburg, August 14, 2001, and MRC, Durban, August 16, 2001.

[71]See, for instance, Benatar, "South Africa's Transition in a Globalizing World," pp. 357–360; "The Cruelest Curse," *The Economist*, February 24, 2001; and "The Limits of $100 Million," *Washington Post*, December 29, 2000.

region can now contemplate their use.[72] Pretoria has been largely unwilling to embrace the widespread adoption of ART programs, however. Although AIDS activists and pediatricians won a landmark ruling in December 2001 forcing the government to provide ARTs to expectant mothers infected with HIV—which has been shown to be an extremely cost-effective method of mitigating mother-child transmission—it remains unclear how comprehensively these drugs will be distributed.[73] The Mbeki administration continues to argue that the effectiveness of ARTs remains unproven and that certain treatments may be toxic to the patient.[74] The President has also made several ill-advised pronouncements alluding to the presumed motives of Western pharmaceutical companies in developing poor countries where up to 50 percent of people do not have access to even the most basic drugs.[75]

At this stage, Pretoria's main response to the epidemic has been to impress prevention and control through abstinence, faithfulness to one partner, and condom use. As part of this effort, ZAR500 million (US$62.5 million) has been invested in educational and awareness programs and more than 200 million condoms have been dispersed.[76] However, these initiatives will have no bearing on the millions of South Africans who have already contracted HIV and who will die over the next five to ten years from AIDS. Moreover, most of the publicity has focused on a U.S.-style "Love Life" billboard campaign, the message of which health workers claim has been largely lost on the bulk of the population because of overly complex and

---

[72]See Brubaker, "The Limits of $100 Million." In large part, the willingness of international pharmaceutical companies to lower the price of ARTs stems from threats made by developing countries to ignore patent laws and allow the manufacture of generic drugs to treat AIDS.

[73]See, for instance, "South Africa Must Dispense AIDS Drug to Pregnant Women," *New York Times*, December 14, 2001.

[74]Although there are legitimate concerns about the toxicity of certain antiretrovirals, especially those used to treat perinatal transmission, the proven benefits of these treatments is generally considered to far outweigh any potential dangers that might ensue.

[75]Author interviews, SABTS, Johannesburg, August 14, 2001, and MRC, Durban, August 16, 2001. See also Benatar, "South Africa's Transition in a Globalizing World," p. 363.

[76]Steyn Speed, "ANC Pamphlet on World AIDS Day," available at http://lists.sn.apc. org/pipermail/election2000/20001201/000082.html.

subtle wording and imaging.[77] It is also worth pointing out that achieving widespread behavioral and attitudinal change will take time (as has been evidenced with antismoking campaigns), something that is likely to be especially true in the case of such basic drives and needs as exist in sexual relations.[78]

One potentially useful development that has occurred was the creation of a National AIDS Council (NAC) in early 2000. Chaired by the Deputy President of South Africa, Jacob Zuma, the council aims to assist in AIDS policy formulation, coordination, information exchange, and programmatic assessment. The value of the NAC stems from its cross-representational membership, which denotes perhaps the most concerted attempt to date to bring together sectoral and technical experts in one overarching forum.[79] At the time of this writing, however, the council had been accorded with neither the budgetary nor the programmatic authority necessary to effectively fulfill its stated mandate.[80]

Nongovernmental Responses

The lack of concerted government action to deal with the HIV/AIDS crisis in South Africa has prompted several other stakeholders to institute policies and initiatives of their own. Notable examples have included

- *Measures precipitated by industry.* Several companies have been instrumental in working with surrounding communities to educate prostitutes on preventative behaviors, such as condom use, with many also offering free screening and HIV/AIDS treatment. A few firms have also begun to pay the full cost of treatment for their employees (though a substantial number are moving to contract labor to offset all responsibility in this regard). The Coca-Cola Foundation, for instance, has stated that it will coordinate the efforts of its sub-Saharan subsidiaries and bottling

---

[77]Author interview, MRC, Durban, August 16, 2001.

[78]Benatar, "South Africa's Transition in a Globalizing World," p. 360.

[79]Whiteside and Sunter, *AIDS*, pp. 126–127.

[80]Author interview, MRC, Durban, August 16, 2001.

partners to support AIDS education, prevention, and treatment programs across the region.[81]

- *Privately backed initiatives.* One of the most important developments that has taken place in this regard is a major health investment drive financed by the Bill and Melinda Gates Foundation. In 2000, the nonprofit organization announced grants in excess of US$90 million to help battle AIDS in Africa. The funds will be used to develop microbicidal treatments for women, train health workers, and provide for children orphaned by AIDS. Recipients of grants in South Africa include the Palliative Medical Institute, the Health Systems Trust, the Planned Parenthood Association of South Africa, and AFRICARE.[82] In January 2001, the Gates Foundation also issued a grant of US$100 million to help support the vaccine development work of the International AIDS Vaccine Initiative and its South African chapter. The pledge has received additional backing from the World Bank as well as the Rockefeller, Sloan, and Starr Foundations.[83]

- *Ad hoc and sector-specific programs.* Two highly visible schemes have been instituted over the last few years, On the Right Track AIDS Train and Trucking Against AIDS. The first, in effect, acts as a moving conference that travels around the country promoting discussion and debate on HIV/AIDS and features delegates from women's organizations, the scientific and academic communities, and the media. The second is a joint project aimed specifically at the road freight industry and promoting awareness about protected sex among long-distance truck drivers. Launched in 2000, the project involves representatives from the Department of Transport, the Road Transport Industry Education and Train-

---

[81]United Nations, "UN Anti-AIDS Effort Enlists Coca-Cola to Curb Spread of Epidemic in Africa," June 21, 2001, available at http://allafrica.com/stories/200106210333.html.

[82]Bill and Melinda Gates Foundation, "The Bill and Melinda Gates Foundation Announces New HIV/AIDS Grants at World AIDS Conference," press release, July 12, 2000, available at http://www.gatesfoundation.org/pressroom/release.asp?Prindex=245.

[83]Bill and Melinda Gates Foundation, "Pledges US$100 Million Toward $550 Million AIDS Vaccine Goal," press release, January 27, 2001, available at http://www.gatesfoundation.org/pressroom/release.asp?Prindex=344.

ing Board, trade unions, and commercial transportation companies (including Engen and Mercedes-Benz).[84]

Although privatized and industrial responses are important, the latitude for them to make a decisive impact on the spread of HIV/AIDS in South Africa has been minimal. As with the NAC, these initiatives have failed to attract support from the central administration and continue to be held captive to the predilections of a government that has so far eschewed a full, open, and constructive debate on the disease and its root causes based on objective evaluations of all available data.[85]

THE INTERNATIONAL RELEVANCE OF THE HIV/AIDS CRISIS IN SOUTH AFRICA

It is readily apparent that the HIV/AIDS crisis in South Africa carries significant consequences for the country's security—economically, militarily, in terms of national crime, and as an issue of basic human survivability. The implications of the epidemic extend well beyond Pretoria's national borders, however, and have direct relevance both regionally and internationally.

South Africa remains crucial to the overall stability of the sub-Saharan region by virtue of its relative wealth, power, size, and status. Not only do neighboring countries depend on Pretoria in terms of trade, investment, and markets, they also look to the republic as the logical state to help dampen and mitigate local sources of tension and conflict. In addition, the republic acts as a crucial diplomatic anchor in Africa, playing the lead role on such bodies as the Southern African Development Community and the Organization of African Unity. Any decisive reduction in South Africa's own security, therefore, is sure to have a highly negative impact on wider regional stability, exacerbating the poverty, internal chaos, and general disruption that have confined countries like Zimbabwe, Zambia, Mozambique,

---

[84]Whiteside and Sunter, *AIDS*, pp. 128–130.

[85]Author interview, MRC, Durban, August 16, 2001.

DRC, Malawi, and Angola to the very lowest echelons of the human development index.[86]

The pandemic also has direct relevance for the wider global community. South Africa remains a reservoir of HIV infection that puts other countries at risk, including, in era of globalization, those with boundaries far from Pretoria's frontline states. Moreover, as noted above, any diminution in the republic's own standing is almost certainly going to exacerbate instability in sub-Saharan Africa. This could well heighten pressure on outside states to undertake a more direct role in the affairs of the region, particularly resource-rich polities that presently rely on Pretoria to act as a viable African conflict dampener and middle power broker (such as the United States and the European Union).[87]

Most significantly, however, the HIV/AIDS crisis in South Africa is a stark reminder of the pervasive and insidious impact that infectious organisms can have on a state's wider stability and viability. Many of the conditions underscoring the spread of HIV—poverty, apathy, urban sprawl, misinformation, lack of public infrastructure, and societal dislocation/imbalance—have relevance to disease incidence in general and exist on a universal basis (albeit in varying degrees). A crisis of similar proportions could, therefore, break out in any country at any time, particularly given an international environment that is at once both global and interdependent in nature.

In short, the South African case underscores, in the most visible terms, the need for national and international disease preparedness. This requirement is as incumbent on the United States as it is on polities in Africa, Asia, Europe, and Latin America, and it is to consideration of this issue that this report turns in Chapters Four and Five.

---

[86]Author interview, London School of Tropical Medicine and Health, London, August 20, 2001. For an explanation of the human development index, see http://www.undp.org/hdro/.

[87]In this sense, if South Africa fails, so does southern Africa. Such considerations have particular relevance for America and European states such as France and Britain (the former by virtue of its role as a global hegemon, the latter due to their historic/colonial ties), as it would then, by default, fall to these countries to "pick up the pieces," not only in South Africa but regionally as well.

Chapter Four

U.S. SECURITY AND THE RISK POSED BY
INFECTIOUS DISEASES

While the average American life expectancy is substantially higher than it was in the past (and continues to grow) and many infectious diseases have been eliminated from the continent over the past century, microorganisms still pose a significant and increasing threat to the country. According to the National Intelligence Council (NIC), "New and reemerging infectious diseases will . . . complicate US and global security over the next 20 years. These diseases will endanger US citizens at home and abroad, threaten armed forces deployed overseas, and exacerbate social and political instability in key countries and regions in which the United States has significant interests."[1] In recognizing the increasing threat posed by infectious disease, the NIC marked a watershed in U.S. foreign policy, particularly in the context of expanding its focus beyond traditional, state-centered sources of instability.

Why are emerging and reemerging infectious diseases on the rise? Many of the factors discussed in Chapter Two regarding the general increased microbial threat apply equally to developing countries and to the United States, including globalization, modern medical practices, accelerating urbanization, global warming, and changing social and behavioral patterns. (Some apply to the United States to a greater extent than others.) This chapter analyzes these various influences in greater detail and delineates the impact that infectious

---

[1]NIC, "The Global Infectious Disease Threat and Its Implications for the United States," p. 5.

disease is currently having on the United States, individually, societally, politically, financially, and strategically.

IMPACT AND SPREAD OF DISEASE IN THE UNITED STATES

Gauging the true impact of infectious disease on the United States is problematic for several reasons. First, the current burden of most infectious illnesses is very low compared with what it might have been had vaccines and other preventative treatments not been used for decades. Second (and related to this), is the fact that the prevalence of pathogenic organisms is liable to increase dramatically in the absence of effective control measures. Third, because of the multiplier effect, every case of disease that is successfully mitigated now reduces future incidence by more than one. Finally, significant intangible costs and effects often surround disease spread and containment, such as social stigmatization, loss of worker productivity, apprehension, grief, and pain.

This being said, there are certain indices that can be used to provide a rough illustration of how infectious ailments are presently serving to affect the United States. In terms of human lives, pathogenic organisms claim approximately 170,000 people annually, which is nearly double the historic low in 1980. Some of the most pervasive killers currently include AIDS, influenza, and foodborne illnesses. Combined, these conditions kill approximately 56,000 people every year (17,000, 30,000, and 9,000, respectively).[2] Certain deaths that have not traditionally been regarded as infectious disease–related, including heart disease and cancer, have also been reclassified as such.[3]

New and existing diseases cross American borders in ever increasing numbers. HIV, West Nile virus, Lyme disease, Legionnaires' disease, hantavirus pulmonary syndrome, and nearly 30 other diseases were first recognized in the latter half of the 20th century in the United

---

[2]NIC, p. 6.

[3]NIC, p. 10. For instance, nearly four million Americans are infected with the hepatitis C virus, which can cause liver cancer and cirrhosis. The death toll may surpass that of AIDS by 2005. Also, the role of human papilloma virus in cancer of the female organs is increasingly being recognized.

States. Multidrug-resistant TB, antibiotic-resistant *Streptococcus pneumoniae* (the bacteria that cause ear infections), pneumonia, meningitis, rabies, and diarrheal disease caused by *Cryptosporidium parvum* and by *E. coli* OH157 all also surged at the end of the 1900s. Underscoring all this is the increased threat of bioterrorism, which has the potential to claim a significant number of lives in a short period of time.

In addition to taking human lives, outbreaks and epidemics cause a considerable amount of chaos and can have a large economic toll. The CDC estimates that the total direct and indirect cost of infectious disease is approximately $120 billion per year.[4] The lifetime, discounted, direct medical outlay of treating a person with HIV alone is thought to be $96,000,[5] while total costs for Lyme disease, if not identified early, can range from $2,228 to $6,724 per patient per year.[6]

The toll wrought by animal infectious disease outbreaks can be just as significant. The U.S. Department of Agriculture (USDA) has estimated that if a hoof-and-mouth disease outbreak occurred in the United States, it could cost the livestock industry $20 billion over 15 years because of increased prices for consumers, reduced agricultural productivity, and restricted trade.[7]

FACTORS AFFECTING THE SCOPE AND SPREAD OF INFECTIOUS DISEASE IN THE UNITED STATES

Despite the costs described above, the impact of disease on America is still manageable. However, this could change rapidly as Americans are exposed daily to growing numbers of new, more virulent, and even common organisms. The reasons are complex and diverse but generally include increased travel and trade, changes in agricultural practice, more promiscuous drug and sex patterns, greater use of

---

[4]NIC, p. 54.

[5]Direct medical costs include physician and clinical staff charges, medications, devices and appliances, and diagnostic tests.

[6]CDC, "Economic Costs for Patient Care from Infectious Diseases, United States," available at http://www.cdc.gov/ncidod/emergplan/box02.htm.

[7]As cited in NIC, p. 58.

antibiotics, use and donation of blood products, climatic change, tainted water supplies, and the increased risk of bioterrorism.

Globalization—Travel, Migration, and Trade

Americans are at increased risk of contracting exotic illnesses from both travel abroad and contact with visitors to the United States. Almost 60 million citizens traveled internationally in 1998. With less than 36 hours of travel time between most parts of the world, many diseases may incubate and emerge only once a person has returned home. In addition, approximately one million immigrants and refugees enter the United States each year, many of whom come from countries burdened by infectious illness.[8] Immigrants entering America for extended stays must undergo medical screening; however, such requirements obviously do not apply to those who enter illegally.[9] Rises in the number of diseases such as TB and malaria have been directly related to these "irregular" foreigners. In 1999, for example, of the more than 150,000 illegal immigrants who were caught and then examined for infections by the U.S. Public Health Service, 126 people were diagnosed with TB. This number is 25 times the number that would be expected if Americans born in the United States were examined and more than four times the numbers that would be expected of the country's foreign-born population.[10] Exacerbating the situation is the fact that many immigrants, both legal and illegal, do not have adequate access to healthcare once they arrive in the United States.[11]

---

[8]NIC, p. 56.

[9] In the 1990s, it is estimated that three to four million undocumented aliens entered the United States. J. S. Passel and M. Fix, "US Immigration at the Beginning of the 21st Century," testimony before the Subcommittee on Immigration and Claims, U.S. House of Representatives, August 2, 2001, available at www.urban.org/TESTIMON/ passel_fix_08-02-01.html, accessed November 9, 2001.

[10]Nick Chiles, "Major Screening for TB Shows Contrast in Conditions Since Days of Ellis Island," *New York Times* online, January 11, 2000, available at http://www. nytimes.com/learning/teachers/featured_articles/20000111tuesday.html, accessed December 15, 2001.

[11]M. Lillie-Blanton and J. Hudman, "Untangling the Web: Race/Ethnicity, Immigration, and the Nation's Health," *American Journal of Public Health*, Vol. 91, No. 11, November 2001, p. 1736.

While laws and border regulations attempt to provide a level of external security from diseases, because of the number of people and goods that enter the United States each year, the likelihood of intercepting an infected person, animal, or plant is very small. The effectiveness of this system of border protection is also open to question. According to the Committee on International Science, Engineering, and Technology (CISET), only about 1 percent of goods entering the country are screened at their point of disembarkation, and notification requirements as described by the Public Health Service Act and Foreign Quarantine Regulations do not cover people who are not obviously ill, animals or insect vectors carrying disease, or those arriving by automobile. The ability of the CDC surveillance regime to identify unfamiliar illnesses entering the country is also debatable, not least because inspectors staff only seven ports of entry.[12] In reality, U.S. defense relies on surveillance at the local rather than federal level. As described in Chapter Five, however, the local public health infrastructure has been neglected over the past quarter century.

Increased animal and food trade has also affected the microbial threat to the United States. The Food Safety and Inspection Service (FSIS) screens food products for an array of zoonotic diseases, including rabies, TB, and brucellosis. However, only a small number of samples are tested and new diseases may not be immediately recognized, potentially exposing humans and animals to deadly infections. Equally, while the USDA's Animal and Plant Health Inspection Service (APHIS) attempts to protect U.S. livestock by excluding and eliminating disease-causing foreign animals, a lack of resources has affected the ability to carry out comprehensive inspections. Indeed, even when contaminated products are detected, the USDA, the Food and Drug Administration (FDA), and other federal agencies have little enforcement power.[13]

---

[12]The seven ports are the airports in New York, Miami, Chicago, Seattle, San Francisco, Los Angeles, and Honolulu. At other ports, airline workers, CDC-contract physicians and Immigration and Naturalization Service officials fill this function. As a result of the paucity of inspections, the CDC invoked its power to detain people at U.S. ports of entry only three times from 1982 to 1992. C. H. Foreman, Jr., *Plagues, Products, and Politics: Emergent Public Health Hazards and National Policymaking,* Washington, D.C.: Brookings Institution Press, 1994, p. 62.

[13]The USDA regulates red meat, poultry, and certain egg products under the Federal Meat Inspection Act and the Poultry Products Inspection Act, while the FDA controls the safety of all other foods under the Federal Food, Drug, and Cosmetic Act (FFDCA).

Increases in trade and shipment of food products, both domestic and foreign, constantly expose individuals to a variety of diseases. According to the NIC, "The globalization of the food supply means that nonhygienic food production, preparation, and handling practices in originating countries can introduce pathogens endangering foreign as well as local populations."[14] In the United States, it is estimated that 76 million people suffer from some sort of foodborne illness each year. Nine of the most serious ailments are listed in Table 4.1.

Table 4.1

Laboratory-Confirmed Cases of Nine Foodborne
Diseases Under Surveillance in the
United States, 2000

Disease	Cases
Salmonellosis	4,640
Campylobacteriosis	4,237
Shigellosis	2,324
E. Coli 0157 infection	631
Cryptosporidiosis	484
Yersiniosis	131
Listeriosis	101
Vibrio infections	61
Cyclospora infections	22

SOURCE: "Preliminary FoodNet Data on the Incidence of Foodborne Illnesses—Selected Sites, United States, 2000," *MMWR Weekly*, Vol. 50, No. 13, April 6, 2001, pp. 241–246, available at http://www.cdc.gov/mmwr/preview/mmwrhtml/mm5013a1.htm, accessed June 21, 2002.

Under the FFDCA, the FDA inspects these products to detect and forbid adulterated or misbranded foods and other products from crossing state borders. The FDA can use limited administrative enforcement tools such as voluntary recalls when violations are found; however, the FDA must rely on the Justice Department to initiate harsher actions such as injunctions, seizures, or prosecutions. *The FDA does not have the power to mandate recalls.* FSIS inspectors, who inspect meat and poultry, also *do not have mandatory recall authority,* and inspectors must go through a federal district court to direct a U.S. marshal to seize product. See Donna U. Vogt, "CRS Issue Brief for Congress: Food Safety Issues in the 106th Congress," February 12, 1999, available at http://www.csa.com/hottopics/ern/99jul/ag-38.html, accessed December 15, 2001.

[14]NIC, p. 22.

Changes in Agricultural Practice

Modern agricultural practices in the United States have also increased the risks from the food supply. Advances in technology— such as antibiotics, automatic feeding, and automatic milking— allow farmers to breed animals in close proximity to one another, which provides a perfect setting for the transmission of viral and bacterial agents. Moreover, the rapidity with which animals are shipped across the country makes it difficult to track the geographic spread of infections. From a public health perspective, this becomes especially problematic in the case of zoonotic diseases. Given the relative ease of transformation from animal to deadly human virus, it would be not be difficult for infections of this type to spread among the U.S. populace where large numbers of immunocompromised animals are shipped cross-country daily.[15]

Behavioral Changes

In the United States, as elsewhere in the world, more permissive sexual behavior and prolific intravenous drug use have opened up new pathways for human-to-human microbial transmission. Many STDs have seen a meteoric rise in the United States since the 1960s due to the sexual revolution, with HIV/AIDS being perhaps the deadliest example of the dangers of these types of behaviors.[16] During the first 20 years of the American HIV/AIDS epidemic, for example, 774,467 persons were reported with AIDS, more than half of whom subsequently died.[17]

---

[15]Recently, scientists at the University of Wisconsin came to understand that there are relatively few genetic steps between the chicken influenza and the human pathogen, raising fears of another outbreak similar to the one in Hong Kong. According to John Oxford, a flu expert and professor of virology at St. Bartholomew's and the Royal London Hospital, "rather small changes in vital places can make the difference between life and death," as quoted in G. Kolata, "Clues to Deadly Virus Changes Seen," *San Jose Mercury News*, September 7, 2001, available at www.mercurycenter.com/cgi-bin/edtoolssss/printpage/printpage_ba.cgi, accessed September 7, 2001.

[16]Mitchell Cohen, "Changing Patterns of Infectious Disease," *Nature*, Vol. 406, 2000, pp. 762–767.

[17]"HIV and AIDS—United States, 1981—2000," *MMWR*, Vol. 50, No. 21, June 1, 2001, pp. 430–434.

Although HIV/AIDS first spread through the relatively open American homosexual community, it is now most often spread among intravenous drug users. According to the CDC, half of all new infections currently result from the sharing of needles to inject heroin and cocaine.[18]

The threat of HIV/AIDS in the United States may also be increasing due to complacency brought on by the success of ARTs. This is especially true among MSMs and in minority populations as indicated by studies of STDs and sexual behaviors.[19] As mentioned elsewhere in Chapter Three, persons infected with HIV/AIDS are at greater risk of contracting and succumbing to many other opportunistic infections that are on the rise, such as TB.[20] The prevalence of drug-resistant microorganisms, discussed below, further complicates treatment of those living with compromised immune systems.

Advances in technology have also influenced behavioral patterns by changing the way Americans live. This has relevance for disease as it brings individuals into contact with a whole new subset of micro-

---

[18]See CDC–National Center for HIV, STD, and TB Prevention–Division of HIV/AIDS Prevention, "HIV/AIDS Surveillance Supplemental Reports," available at http://www.cdc.gov/hiv/stats/hasrsupp51.htm. See also S. D. Holmberg, "The Estimated Prevalence and Incidence of HIV in 96 Large US Metropolitan Areas," *American Journal of Public Health*, Vol. 86, No. 5, 1996, pp. 642–654. It should be noted that many commentators reject the idea that it is possible to "map" the number and pattern of new HIV infections. See, for instance, the Committee on HIV Prevention Strategies in the United States, *No Time to Lose: Getting More From HIV Prevention*, Washington D.C.: The Institute of Medicine, 2001.

[19]From 1998 through 2000 a study Phase II of the Young Men's Study was performed and sampled male-to-male sex with partners of ages 23 to 29 in six U.S. cities. Preliminary data showed that 13 percent of 3,000 men were HIV-positive, with prevalence rates of 7 percent among whites, 14 percent among Hispanics, and 32 percent among blacks. In a recent study of young men, high HIV incidence was associated with having more than five male sex partners during the preceding six months, having unprotected anal sex with men, or having injected drugs. "HIV Incidence Among Young Men Who Have Sex With Men—Seven US Cities, 1994–2000," *MMWR*, Vol. 50, No. 21, 2001, pp. 440–444.

[20]In addition to HIV/AIDS, improvements in healthcare and disease treatment have led to a significant increase in the number of immunocompromised people in the United States. The growing elderly population, patients undergoing chemotherapy, and those taking immunosuppressive drugs (such as transplant patients) are all at increased risk for contracting and succumbing to infectious diseases. These individuals also put the greater population at risk because they can become carriers of many illnesses.

organisms. For instance, water towers used for climatic control provide highly suitable breeding grounds for *L. pneumophila*.[21] Equally, while the use of refrigeration to extend the life of foods has reduced exposure to many bacteria, it also led to the rise of organisms, such as *Listeria monocytogenes*, that thrive in colder environments. (*L. monocytogenes* causes nearly 2,000 illnesses and more than 400 deaths per year in the United States.) It is often difficult to predict how technological advances and associated behavioral changes will affect the balance between humans and microorganisms.

Misuse of Antibiotics and Other Medicines

Overuse of antibiotics and other drugs in the United States to "treat" viruses together with failure to finish prescriptions and the use of antibiotics in animals have dramatically hurt the effectiveness of these medications and led to the rapid rise of highly resistant "supergerms."[22] According to the CDC, nearly all bacteria of concern have developed some degree of resistance in part because of the fact that up to 50 million prescriptions a year are written for antibiotics unnecessarily.[23] For instance, according to the National Institute of Allergy and Infectious Diseases (NIAID), drug resistance is a factor in the threat posed by TB, gonorrhea, malaria, and pneumococcal diseases. Treating these hardy microbes has a high cost as well, perhaps

---

[21]This was first recognized in 1976 when pneumonia struck 221 people at an American Legion convention in Philadelphia.

[22]For a full discussion of antibiotic resistance, see S. B. Levy, *The Antibiotic Paradox: How the Misuse of Antibiotics Destroys Their Curative Powers*, 2nd edition, Cambridge, Mass.: Perseus Publishing, 2002; Laurie Garrett, *The Coming Plague: Newly Emerging Diseases in a World out of Balance*, New York: Penguin Books, 1994; WHO, *Overcoming Antimicrobial Resistance*, 2000, available at www.who.int/infectious-disease-report/; Stuart B. Levy, "The Challenge of Antibiotic Resistance," *Scientific American*, Vol. 278, No. 3, March 1998, pp. 46–53; and B. Schwartz, D. Bell, J. M. Hughes, "Preventing the Emergence of Antimicrobial Resistance: A Call for Action by Clinicians, Public Health Officials, and Patients," *JAMA*, Vol. 278, No. 11, September 17, 1997, pp. 901–904.

[23]CDC, "Antibiotic Resistance," available at http://www.cdc.gov/antibiotic resistance/, accessed June 21, 2002, and CNN, "Antibiotic Resistance a Growing Threat," June 12, 2000, available at http://www.cnn.com/2000/health/06/12/anti biotic.resistance, accessed June 21, 2002, report improper drug use to blame for the growing resistance.

as much as $30 billion per year in the United States.[24] Hardly any new antibiotics have been developed, with only one additional antibiotic class introduced in the country during the past 15 years.[25]

In the United States, antibiotic-resistant, nosocomial (hospital-acquired) infections caused by resistant *S. aureus* currently kill approximately 14,000 patients annually.[26] Generally up to 70 percent of hospital-acquired infections are caused by drug-resistant microbes.

Overall the numbers of resistant organisms are rising. More than 50 percent of all TB cases in the United States are now "immune" to at least one drug, and 32 percent were resistant to two or more of the premier anti-TB drugs in 1994, up from 10 percent in 1984.[27]

Donated Blood Products

Another aspect of U.S. medical practice that can potentially spread dangerous diseases is the use of donated blood products. The nation's blood supply, while strictly regulated and screened, can be protected only from readily identified pathogens. Essentially this means that diseases like HIV, hepatitis C, and variant Creutzfeldt-Jakob, which have long incubation periods, could be spread through the blood supply before they become immediately apparent.

---

[24]NIAID, "Antimicrobial Resistance," fact sheet, available at http://www.niaid.nih.gov/factsheets/antimicro.htm, accessed January 16, 2002.

[25]Overuse and misuse of fungal and viral treatments contribute to the dangers of microbes as well. Aventis Pharmaceuticals, Inc., introduced SYNERCID and Pharmacia & Upjohn introduced Zyvox in 2000 to treat gram-positive infections such as pneumonia and bacteremia (CNN, "FDA Approves First in a Long-Awaited New Class of Antibiotics," April 18, 2000, available at www.cnn.co/2000/HEALTH/04/18/new.antibiotic, accessed December 7, 2000).

[26] In excess of 80 percent of *S. aureus* isolates in the United States are penicillin resistant and 32 percent are methicillin resistant (NIC, p. 6). More generally, it is estimated that nosocomial infections contributed to nearly 90,000 deaths in 1995 and cost $4.5 billion. See Robert Weinstein, "Nosocomial Infection Update," *Emerging Infectious Diseases*, Vol. 4, No. 3, 1998, available at http://www.cdc.gov/ncidod/eid/vol4no3/weinstein.htm, accessed December 7, 2000.

[27]NIC, p. 55. An additional factor that played a role in exacerbating the challenge in dealing with TB during the 1980s was the abandonment of the surveillance system for recognizing multidrug-resistant TB strains. This was reinstated in 1993, however, once it was recognized that cases of resistance TB were once again rising.

The latent dangers of covert pathogenic transmission are well illustrated by hepatitis C. Although Harvey Alter, a researcher at the National Institutes of Health (NIH), had first recognized in the 1970s that a new form of hepatitis was attacking livers of blood recipients, it was not until 1989 that Michael Houghton at Chiron Corporation identified the etiologic agent—hepatitis C virus. Consequently, for almost 20 years patients in the United States and elsewhere were at about a 30 percent risk of receiving blood contaminated by hepatitis C. This particular disease has proven especially problematic to fight because until recently researchers have been unable to grow it in the laboratory. Moreover, the causative viral agent mutates often, making it difficult for the human body to develop full immunity after exposure. Currently, nearly three million Americans are living with chronic hepatitis C infection, about 10 to 20 percent of whom may develop liver-destroying cirrhosis or cancer.[28]   HIV also contaminated the blood supply prior to 1985 when screening was initiated; however, this has had a less devastating effect on the population, resulting in just over 1,000 AIDS cases at its peak in 1993.[29]

Climatic Change

Climatic change has also provided a mechanism for escalating the exposure of individual Americans to new and more virulent pathogens. As noted in Chapter Two, increasing evidence suggests that disturbances in climate and weather patterns play a significant role in influencing the distribution media for infectious pathogenic agents.[30] In the short term, they can increase vector populations that spread disease to human hosts. For example, the New Mexico hantavirus pulmonary syndrome outbreak that emerged in 1993 occurred after an unusually wet spring in the Southwest, which allowed the deer mouse carrier population to swell dramatically; by 1995, the disease had spread to 21 U.S. states.[31] In the long term, if climatic

---

[28]Charlene Crabb, "Hard-Won Advances Spark Excitement About Hepatitis C," *Science,* Vol. 294, 2001, pp. 506–507.

[29]"HIV and AIDS—1981–2000," *MMWR*, pp. 430–434.

[30]Paul Epstein, "Climate and Health," *Science*, Vol. 285, 1999, pp. 347–348.

[31]Brian Hjelle, "Hantaviruses, with Emphasis on Four Corners Hantavirus," 1996, available at http://www.bocklabs.wisc.edu/ed/hanta.html, accessed November 16, 2001.

changes are significantly in concert with the introduction of new disease vectors from foreign countries, it is conceivable that infections such as malaria, cholera, and dengue could reestablish themselves in the United States as well as elsewhere.

Tainted Water Supplies

Most of the U.S. water supply is screened only for representative bacteria such as fecal coliforms. This leaves the population at risk from new or unusual pathogens that enter water systems undetected. Moreover, an aging infrastructure has significantly undermined the ability of authorities to ensure that known contaminants are properly removed.[32]

The large and growing population of immunocompromised individuals in the United States increases the significance of water supply contamination. The cryptosporidiosis outbreak in April 1993 in Milwaukee is an example of how extensive the problem can be. In this instance, over 400,000 people became ill and approximately 100 died after the filtration system in the water treatment plant failed. It is certainly possible that another unannounced pathogen could similarly sicken and injure unsuspecting citizens.

Bioterrorism

The spate of anthrax mailings unleashed throughout the United States in fall 2001 transformed the threat of bioterrorism into a reality. Although the human impact (in terms of lost lives) of this manifestation of the disease threat remains tiny in comparison to that of naturally occurring infections, the economic and psychological toll is significant. The U.S. Postal Service alone estimates that the cost of responding to the anthrax attacks as well as new sterilization pro-

---

[32]In February 2001, the Environmental Protection Agency estimated that nearly $151 billion is required over the next 20 years to maintain, replace, and upgrade the water supply system to ensure safe drinking water, with a quarter of these funds dedicated to treatment (U.S. Senate, testimony of Tracy Mehan, Assistant Administrator for Water, U.S. Environmental Protection Agency, before the Committee on Environment and Public Works, Subcommittee on Fisheries, Wildlife, and Water, October 31, 2001, available at http://www.win-water.org/win_legislative/win_testimony/103101mehan. html, accessed November 30, 2001).

cedures for mail will be in the range of $5 billion; this is from an attack in which only five deaths and 17 known infections occurred from a noncontagious disease.[33] The overall human and economic ramifications would be much greater with a contagious weapon.

Public health and medical experts, policymakers and others with genuine or economic motives have undoubtedly fueled the fear of bioterrorism in the United States.[34] However, alarming scientific and psychological changes are occurring, which may increase the overall risk of deliberately introduced diseases. For instance, scientists working to sterilize mice for the purpose of controlling the rodent population have created an extremely virulent mousepox with a technique that might be useful for creating an extremely potent smallpox weapon.[35] Further, in 1997, Russian scientists created a genetically engineered *Bacillus anthracis* (the microbe that causes anthrax) that could overcome protection given by the vaccine currently produced in the United States.[36]

As this chapter shows, the threat of infectious diseases is omnipresent in the United States. This is problematic largely because, just as American citizens are coming into increased contact with emerging and reemerging pathogens, the country's ability to respond to microbial agents has been eroded in many areas. Chapter Five turns

---

[33]WEVA, "US Post Office Acquires Irradiation Technology," October 28, 2001, available at http://www.weva.com/cgi-bin/newsreader.pl?storyid=255&type=I; Ray Schmid, "Post Office Turns to Congress for Financial Help," Associated Press, November 8, 2001, available at http://sns.kcpq.com/sns-anthrax-mail.story.

[34]However, the large-scale use of these weapons by terrorists is unlikely in the near future, because of lack of both motive and technical capabilities. Advisory Panel to Assess Domestic Response Capabilities for Terrorism Involving Weapons of Mass Destruction, *First Annual Report to the President and the Congress—I: Assessing the Threat,* Santa Monica, Calif.: RAND, December 15, 1999; Bruce Hoffman, "Twenty-First Century Terrorism," foreword in James M. Smith and William C. Thomas, eds., *The Terrorism Threat and the U.S. Government Response: Operational and Organizational Factors,* Colorado Springs, Colo.: U.S. Air Force Institute for National Security Studies, 2001.

[35]Ronald J. Jackson et al., "Expression of Mouse Interleukin-4 by a Recombinant Ectromelia Virus Suppresses Cytolytic Lymphocyte Responses and Overcomes Genetic Resistance to Mousepox," *Journal of Virology,* Vol. 75, No. 3, February 2001, pp. 1205–1210.

[36]A. P. Pomerantsev et al., "Expression of Cereolysine AB Genes in Bacillus Anthracis Vaccine Strain Ensures Protection Against Experimental Hemolytic Anthrax Infection," *Vaccine,* Vol. 15, Nos. 17–18, December 1997, pp. 1846–1850.

to this issue, first examining the critical components of U.S. disease prevention and mitigation and then assessing the main gaps that are currently serving to undermine the effectiveness of this overall system.

Chapter Five

U.S. CAPABILITIES TO COUNTER
INFECTIOUS DISEASES

In 1992, the Institute of Medicine (IOM) challenged the United States to respond to the threat of infectious diseases by improving public health and medical capacity. Partly in response to the IOM, in 1994 the CDC drafted a strategy that included improvements in surveillance, applied research, prevention and control, and infrastructure.[1] Recognizing the ongoing risks of increasing global interdependencies, in 1995 the National Science and Technology Council's CISET further recommended that the United States play a stronger role in global efforts to control infectious disease.[2] The CISET report served as the basis for a 1996 Presidential Decision Directive calling for the formation of an emerging infectious disease task force to oversee efforts to develop a global surveillance and response network, enhance research and training, and strengthen cooperation with international partners.[3] The continued emergence of new strains of infectious diseases, changes in healthcare delivery, and new technologies and scientific findings prompted additional action by the

---

[1]CDC, "Preventing Emerging Infectious Diseases," p. 3; CDC, "Addressing Emerging Infectious Disease Threats: A Prevention Strategy for the United States," Atlanta: CDC, 1994.

[2]National Science and Technology Council, *Infectious Disease,* September 1995, available at http://clinton4.nara.gov/textonly/WH/EOP/OSTP/CISET/html/toc.html as "Global Microbial Threats in the 1990s," accessed August 17, 2001.

[3]See The White House, Office of Science and Technology Policy, "Addressing the Threat of Emerging Infectious Diseases," PDD/NSTC-7, June 12, 1996, available at http://www.state.gov/www/global/oes/health/task_force/whthreat.html, accessed June 28, 2001.

CDC, which revised its strategic plan in 1998.[4] Despite these initiatives, however, in 2002 the public health infrastructure across the United States remains variable and in many cases inadequate.

This chapter analyzes U.S. capabilities to counter infectious disease and discusses the challenges posed by this system for maintaining or increasing America's relative success with respect to fighting contagion. The first section assesses efforts by the federal government, particularly the CDC, to bolster state and local capabilities to detect and investigate disease outbreaks and examines legal restrictions to federal action. The second section considers various federal interagency initiatives aimed at addressing foodborne disease, antibiotic resistance, bioterrorism, research, and global surveillance. The final section examines the holes in these systems and the risks inherent in failing to deal with these gaps.

RESOURCES FOR FIGHTING INFECTIOUS DISEASE

In the United States, resources and responsibilities for monitoring, preventing, and controlling infectious disease are distributed throughout the public health system. Hospitals, clinical laboratories, pharmaceutical companies, healthcare providers, universities, and research groups form part of a larger system that works to reduce the impact of pathogens. The CDC acts as the lead U.S. federal agency, providing information, recommendations, and technical assistance in support of state and local public health departments.[5] Although lacking specific authority for public health functions—which remain a state responsibility in the American federal system—this agency assumes the primary burden of surveillance for and initial response to outbreaks.[6] This being said, the actual mobilization of federal resources in response to an outbreak is necessarily contingent on state capabilities to detect problems and request assistance. More-

---

[4]CDC, "Preventing Emerging Infectious Diseases."

[5]Foreman, *Plagues, Products, and Politics,* p. 25.

[6]IOM, "Public Health Systems and Emerging Infections: Assessing the Capabilities of the Public and Private Sectors, Workshop Summary," Washington, D.C.: National Academy Press, 2000, p. 31.

over, the disease mitigation resources that are often contributed at the local level are considerable and should not be ignored.[7]

State and local public health capabilities are coordinated and largely provided for through the CDC, which has recently enhanced its efforts to build capacity in the areas of disease surveillance, investigation, and prevention and control of infectious diseases.[8]

Surveillance and Detection

Surveillance is a core public health function, representing the first link in a chain of activities aimed at countering infectious viral and bacterial agents.[9] Disease surveillance in the United States hinges on a staged process of reporting from clinicians and laboratories to local or state health departments to the CDC. Although the CDC represents the pinnacle of this system, statutory authority for disease surveillance mechanisms and the determination of associated monitoring agendas belongs to states and their respective environmental and public health departments.[10]

---

[7]Foreman, *Plagues, Products, and Politics,* p. 44. Foreman cites officials of the CDC's Epidemiology Program Office to the effect that the CDC may initiate investigations in the case of multistate outbreaks.

[8]In FY 2002, the CDC invested $332 million to fight diseases, a portion of which is specifically earmarked for assistance to states and localities. It should be noted, however, that for FY 2002 HIV/AIDS, STD, and TB prevention are budgeted separately for over $1 billion. The same is true for immunization, bioterrorism, and surveillance, which are slated for nearly $600 million, $182 million, and $27 million, respectively. All of the recommended funding represents increases from the previous year's budget with the exception of surveillance, according to the U.S. Department of Health and Human Services, "FY 2002 President's Budget for HHS," p. 33, available at http://www.hhs.gov/budget/pdf/h.PDF, accessed August 30, 2001; also see ASM Clinical Microbiology Issues Update, "ASM Submits Testimony to Congress," April 2001, available at http://www.asmusa.org/pasrc/clinicalmicro-april2001.htm, accessed June 22, 2002.

[9]The CDC defines public health surveillance as "the ongoing, systematic collection, analysis, interpretation, and dissemination of health data, including information on clinical diagnoses, laboratory-based diagnoses, specific syndromes, health-related behaviors, and use of products related to health." GAO, "Global Health: Framework for Infectious Disease Surveillance," GAO/NSIAD-00-205R, July 20, 2000, pp. 5–6; CDC, "Preventing Emerging Infectious Diseases," p. 17.

[10]At the state level, epidemiologists analyze test results and laboratory reports, initiate epidemiological investigations, and design, institute, and evaluate prevention and

An epidemic may be detected by routine surveillance or by the recognition of an unusual cluster of cases, often by an alert clinician. Sometimes this involves the reporting of cases and symptoms not under formal surveillance. This occurred with the hantavirus outbreak in the Southwest in 1993 (see Chapter Four), when two deaths from sudden respiratory failure prompted a U.S. Indian Health Service physician to alert the New Mexico state health department, which in turn called in the CDC.[11] Similarly, the investigation that revealed the presence of West Nile virus in the Western Hemisphere was instigated by a hospital infectious disease specialist who reported unusual cases of suspected encephalitis or meningitis to the New York City Department of Health.[12]

The bulk of routine surveillance reporting from states to the CDC is conducted under the auspices of the National Notifiable Disease Surveillance System (NNDSS, see the Appendix).[13] State disease reporting to CDC, however, is voluntary. Reflecting this, only 60 percent of the 19 notifiable diseases on the national list were reported in more than 90 percent of U.S. states and territories in January 1999.[14] In an effort to enhance the effectiveness of the overall U.S. disease monitoring regime, the CDC is currently in the process of developing the National Electronic Disease Surveillance System (NEDSS), the goal of which is to coordinate, and thus improve, local, state, and national surveillance systems (see the Appendix).[15] In addition, the

---

control measures. GAO, "Emerging Infectious Diseases: National Surveillance System Could Be Strengthened," GAO/T-HEHS-99-62, February 25, 1999, p. 4.

[11]Stephen S. Morse, "Controlling Infectious Diseases," Federation of American Scientists, available at http://www.fas.org/promed/papers/morse.htm, accessed July 11, 2001.

[12]GAO, "West Nile Virus Outbreak: Lessons for Public Health Preparedness," GAO/HEHS-00-180, September 2000, p. 10.

[13]Incidence of diseases deemed notifiable by the CDC and a given state are reported to the CDC on a weekly basis and published in the *Morbidity and Mortality Weekly Report* (MMWR). The National Electronic Telecommunications System for Surveillance was established in 1985 to facilitate weekly computer-based reporting of surveillance data from state health departments to the CDC.

[14]Sandra Roush et al., "Mandatory Reporting of Diseases and Conditions by Health Care Professionals and Laboratories," *JAMA*, Vol. 282, No. 2, July 14, 1999, pp. 165–168.

[15]CDC, "Supporting Public Health Surveillance through the National Electronic Disease Surveillance System (NEDSS)" available at http://www.cdc.gov/od/hissb/docs/NEDSS%20Intro.pdf, accessed July 6, 2001.

CDC is working to augment epidemiology and laboratory capacity,[16] develop a network for population-based surveillance and research,[17] and establish four provider-based sentinel networks designed to monitor conditions not covered by routine health department surveillance.[18]

Because other surveillance methods often do not provide anything near real-time reporting, and since this is critical for the timely recognition and treatment of infectious outbreaks, there is growing interest in early warnings through syndromic surveillance. This particular type of monitoring relies on reports about syndromes or symptoms that may indicate an epidemic sooner than reports of specific diagnoses.[19] As an example, New York City has established a sentinel network of 11 hospitals that report daily to the New York City Department of Health on the number of hospital admissions via the emergency department.[20]

The Department of Defense (DoD) is developing several other syndromic surveillance systems. The Early Warning Outbreak Recognition System (EWORS), instituted jointly by the U.S. Navy, the Indonesian Ministry of Health, and the WHO, collects daily clinical data from five sentinel sites around Indonesia. Another initiative, the

---

[16]The CDC created the Epidemiology and Laboratory Capacity (ELC) program, and ELC cooperative agreements have been concluded in all 50 states. Funding is also provided to ELC programs in six large local health departments and the territory of Puerto Rico. The average grant award in FY 2000 was $311,000, a portion of which was used to hire 60 epidemiologists and 43 microbiologists.

[17]The Emerging Infection Program (EIP) aims to assess both the public health impact of emerging infections and the measures used to prevent and control them.

[18]Ann Marie Kimball, "Overview and Surveillance of Emerging Infections," available at http://cer.hs.washington.edu/em_inf/emerging/emerg.html, accessed September 3, 2001. Kimball observes that syndromic surveillance is less specific than traditional disease surveillance, and points to the danger that it may supersede laboratory-based surveillance.

[19]Ibid.

[20]Amy E. Smithson and Leslie-Anne Levy, *Ataxia: The Chemical and Biological Terrorism Threat and the U.S. Response,* Stimson Center Report N. 35, available at www.stimson.org/cbw/pubs.cfm?cd=12, p. 256. According to Smithson and Levy, public health officials are considering monitoring other kinds of information that may indicate an outbreak, such as school absenteeism, sick calls to health clinics for certain city employees such as firefighters and police, calls to healthcare hotlines, and sales of drugs to treat flu-like systems.

Global Emerging Infections Surveillance and Response System (GEIS), administers a syndromic surveillance system in the Washington, D.C., area, which records and compares to trends, the outpatient diagnoses in eight syndrome categories from area military medical treatment facilities.[21] Additional information on this system can be found in the Appendix.

Investigation

Once a potential epidemic has been detected, an investigation is necessary to confirm the outbreak, identify the source of infection, and determine its mode of transmission. Investigations may include epidemiological, laboratory, and environmental assessments.[22] The CDC assists state and local health officials, epidemiologists, and laboratory personnel with outbreak investigations by providing technical advice, reference and diagnostic services, and, upon state request, a member of the Epidemic Intelligence Service (EIS) to support field investigations.[23] State and local outbreak investigators may additionally take advantage of Epi-Info and Epi-Map, two public-domain software packages designed by the CDC as standard investigative tools.[24] The CDC also assists state and local public health laboratories through consultation, training, technology transfer, and reference and diagnostic services. The CDC's National Center for Infectious Disease plays an important role in this regard, providing

---

[21]Col. Patrick Kelley, "Bioterrorism: Alert and Response," available at http://cer.hs. washington.edu/em_inf/bio/bio.html, accessed August 31, 2001. Following the attacks on the World Trade Center and Pentagon on September 11, the GEIS system was expanded to worldwide operations.

[22]IOM, "Public Health Systems and Emerging Infections," p. 34. For an interesting and widely acclaimed study on shoe-leather epidemiology, see Arthur Reingold, "Outbreak Investigations—A Perspective," *Emerging Infectious Diseases*, Vol. 4, No. 1, January–March 1998, available at http://www.cdc.gov/ncidod/EID/vol4no1/reingold. htm.

[23]In FY 2000, EIS officers participated in 74 Epidemiologic Assistances (EPI-AIDs), of which 63 were domestic. CDC, "Requests for Epidemiologic Assistance (EPI-AIDs)," available at http://www.cdc.gov/programs/partners9.htm, accessed August 15, 2001.

[24]CDC, "About Epi-Info," available at http://www.cdc.gov/epiinfo/aboutepi.htm, accessed July 12, 2001.

public health laboratories with a reliable supply of microbiological references and working reagents not commercially available.[25]

Currently, there is no comprehensive national laboratory system to support these facilities, with most laboratories cooperating according to local arrangements based on diagnostic capabilities.[26] There are roughly 150,000 physician office and health clinic laboratories, 17,000 independent and hospital laboratories, and 2,000 public health laboratories in the United States.[27] Most of these laboratories also rely on out-of-state or private testing rather than analyses performed by designated state public health facilities.[28] According to Dr. Patty Quinlisk, the CDC provides resources to revamp the public health system's state laboratories, and most if not all laboratories are in the midst of improving their capacity for rapid diagnoses, identification, and coordination.[29]

---

[25]CDC, "National Center for Infectious Disease (HCR)," available at http://www.cdc.gov/maso/ncidfs.htm, accessed August 3, 2001.

[26]Michael R. Skeel, "Toward a National Laboratory System for Public Health," *Emerging Infectious Diseases*, Vol. 7, No. 3, Supplement, June 2001, p. 531. It should be noted, however, that the Division of Laboratory Systems within the CDC's Public Health Practice Program Office is supporting efforts to establish a National Laboratory System, drawing on funding from bioterrorism, food safety, and emerging infectious diseases initiatives. See Division of Laboratory Systems, available at http://www.phppo.cdc.gov/mlp/nls.asp, accessed August 13, 2001.

[27]CDC, "Towards a National Laboratory System," November 2000, p. 3, available at http://www.phppo.cdc.gov/mlp/pdf/nls/nls.1101.pdf, accessed August 3, 2001. With respect to state, local, and territorial public health laboratories, this report adds, "[W]e do not have an accurate estimate of either the number of laboratories in each category or the types and volumes of the important public health testing that they perform."

[28]GAO, "Emerging Infectious Diseases: Consensus on Needed Laboratory Capacity Could Strengthen Surveillance," GAO/HEHS-99-26, February 1999, p. 7.

[29]Author interview with Patty Quinlisk, October 4, 2001. State laboratories may be categorized as belonging to one of three biosafety levels (BSL 2–4). Most clinical laboratories are categorized as BSL-2, while most state public health department labs operate at BSL-3. There are only four BSL-4 laboratories in the United States and no BSL-4 veterinary labs. There are fewer than 20 veterinary laboratories with BSL-3 capabilities. The four labs are located at the CDC in Atlanta, Georgia; the U.S. Army Medical Research Institute of Infectious Disease (USAMRIID) at Fort Detrick, Frederick, Maryland; the NIH Maximum Containment Lab, Bethesda, Maryland; and the Southwest Foundation for Biomedical Research, San Antonio, Texas, according to the American Society for Microbiology, "List of Currently Known BSL-4 Facilities Worldwide," available at http://www.asmusa.org/memonly/asmnews/nov99/figs/t1f1.htm, accessed July 12, 2001.

A number of measures have also been initiated to deal with the specific threat of bioterrorism. One of the most important is a CDC-run program that aims to build capacity for identifying and containing critical biological agents that could be used as weapons. The CDC has also collaborated with the American Society for Microbiology to devise simple screening algorithms for five high-priority bioterrorism agents, and more protocols are under development.[30] In 1999, the CDC trained some 700 laboratory and public health personnel on protocols for detecting, handling, and shipping critical biological agents, and 43 states received CDC funding to improve diagnostic and reference testing capabilities for selected agents.[31] An important feature of these various initiatives is the CDC's Rapid Response and Advanced Technology (RRAT) Laboratory. This lab operates 24 hours a day and is designed to provide diagnostic confirmatory and consultation support for bioterrorism response teams as well as to expedite molecular characterization of critical biological agents in federal BSL-4 facilities.[32] During FY 2000, enhanced diagnostic capabilities for the analysis of tularemia, plague, and anthrax were instituted under the rubric of RRAT.[33]

Additionally, the CDC has been actively engaged in supporting the development of more effective bioterrorist diagnostic capabilities at the state and local levels. An important component of this effort, which has been undertaken in conjunction with the Association of Public Health Laboratories (APHL), is the National Laboratory Training Network. This particular initiative trains public health workers on protocols for screening potential bioterrorism agents, including *B. anthracis, Brucella abortus, Francisella tularensis* and *Yersinia pestis.* The long-term objective is to provide a national sys-

---

[30]James W. Snyder and William Check, *Bioterrorism Threats to Our Future: The Role of the Clinical Microbiology Laboratory in Detection, Identification and Confirmation of Biological Agents*, Washington, D.C.: American Academy of Microbiology, 2001, p. 8.

[31]Gregory D. Koblentz, "Overview of Federal Programs to Enhance State and Local Preparedness for Terrorism with Weapons of Mass Destruction," Belfer Center for Science and International Affairs, Discussion Paper 2001-5, Executive Session on Domestic Preparedness Discussion Paper ESDP-2001-3, Cambridge, Mass.: John F. Kennedy School of Government, Harvard University, April 2001, pp. 19–20.

[32]Koblentz, "Overview of Federal Programs," p. 39.

[33]Comments made by Scott Lillibridge during the ICEID, Atlanta, July 16–19, 2001.

tem for effectively disseminating emergency information and testing guidelines.[34]

Response (Prevention and Control)

The response to an infectious disease epidemic will depend on the disease and circumstances of the outbreak. Prevention and control efforts often involve simple means to interrupt the transmission process of an infectious agent. These measures may take a variety of forms, such as vaccination, rodent or insect (vector) control, food recall, isolation, and quarantine. Because behavior is an important factor in the transmission of most infectious agents, education and information campaigns are also a feature of most disease-response initiatives.

One of the foremost tools in preventing infectious diseases is immunization, which during the last century has eradicated smallpox, eliminated polio from the Americas, and brought measles, rubella, diphtheria, tetanus, *Haemophilus influenzae* type b, and other diseases under control.[35] The National Immunization Program assists health departments in planning, developing, and implementing regular immunization programs and supports the establishment of vaccine supply contracts for the distribution of vaccines to states and localities.[36] The CDC may also provide vaccines or available treatments if there are shortages, usually by supplying state or local health agencies.[37] In addition, CDC's Vaccines for Children program, initiated in 1994, provides free vaccines to public and private providers in all states and territories, with the aim of ensuring immunization of eligible children.[38]

---

[34]CDC, 2001 Program Review, "National Laboratory Network," press kit, available at www.cdc.gov/od/oc/media/presskit/training.htm, pp. 21–22.

[35]"Ten Great Public Health Achievements, 1900–1999," *MMWR,* available at http:// www.cdc.gov/od/nvpo/arttop10.htm, accessed October 15, 2001.

[36]CDC, "About NIP," available at www.cdc.gov/nip/about/, accessed August 15, 2001.

[37]Foreman, *Plagues, Products, and Politics,* p. 74.

[38]Through this program, VFC vaccines are available to children from birth through 18 years old who are eligible for Medicaid, have no health insurance, are Native American or Alaska Native, or have health insurance that does not cover immunizations, provided they go to a federally qualified health center. CDC, "National Immunization

The CDC supports a variety of new and existing community-based programs for generally preventing and controlling diseases, such as the HIV Prevention Community Planning project.[39] The CDC also develops, evaluates, and updates clinical and public health guidelines for a variety of diseases and conditions, most of which can be accessed by state and local health officials via the CDC's online Prevention Guidelines database.[40] Finally, the CDC provides scientific support to the Task Force on Community Preventive Services, an independent group charged with developing recommendations on population-based interventions to prevent disease, injury, and premature death.[41]

While most disease prevention-and-control efforts are generally accepted as necessary for the public good, model legislation financed by the CDC for responding to bioterrorist attacks has come under some fire. Known officially as the Model Emergency Health Powers Act, this statute invests state governors and health officials with broad powers to examine, quarantine, and vaccinate American citizens exposed to pathogenic agents during a major health emergency. Although no state has formally acceded to the plan, the American Legislative Exchange Council, a bipartisan group of state legislators, has warned that the plan would intrude on Americans' civil liberties and could be used for purposes that extend well beyond bioterrorism.[42] Experts reject these arguments, however, and insist that the model law is essential in providing state authorities with the neces-

---

Program: Vaccines for Children," available at http://www.cdc.gov/nip/vfc/Parent/ParentHomePage.htm, accessed August 27, 2001.

[39]CDC, "Preventing Emerging Infectious Diseases," p. 42.

[40]CDC, "Prevention Guidelines," available at http://wonder.cdc.gov/wonder/prevguid/library/library.asp, accessed August 15, 2001.

[41]CDC, "Guide to Community Preventive Services," available at http://www.cdc.gov/programs/partners4.htm, accessed August 15, 2001.

[42]The model legislation, for instance, also gives state authorities the power to "control, restrict and regulate food, fuel, clothing and other commodities, alcoholic beverages, firearms, explosives, and combustibles." See Dave Ebhert, "Model State Bioterror Law Stirs Controversy," Vaccine Information Center, January 3, 2002, available at http://www.vaclib.org/legal/invol.htm. (For the full text of the model law, see http://www.publichealthlaw.net.)

sary statutory authority to act decisively in the event of a bioterrorist attack or emerging infectious disease outbreak.[43]

OTHER FEDERAL PROGRAMS AND INTERAGENCY INITIATIVES

In addition to the state- and local-level counterdisease activities outlined above, various agencies within the federal government work with the CDC and local and international partners to address specific concerns related to infectious disease. This section examines these efforts with respect to foodborne illness, antimicrobial resistance, bioterrorism, research, and global surveillance.

Foodborne Disease

Foodborne illness in the United States has recently received increasing attention. As regulatory agencies, the USDA's FSIS and the FDA play important roles in preventing and responding to outbreaks of foodborne diseases.[44]

In 1996, FSIS issued its rule on Pathogen Reduction and Hazard Analysis and Critical Control Point (HACCP) systems, which mandated the implementation of HACCP systems in meat and poultry facilities. This regulation requires hazard analysis to identify critical points in the food production process and the application of preventive and corrective measures aimed at eliminating hazards at those

---

[43]See, for instance, Marsha Berry and Lawrence Gostin, "Model Emergency Health Powers Act in Response to Bioterrorism Written for the CDC and Governors: Act to Help Ensure Rapid and Orderly Response to Public Health Threats," Georgetown University Law Center, October 30, 2001, available at http://www.law.georgetown.edu/topics/releases/october.30.2001.html.

[44]FSIS is responsible for meat, poultry, and eggs, while the FDA is responsible for all other food products. Currently, FSIS and FDA do not have authority to order mandatory recalls of dangerous food products. The FDA may suggest that a recall is in order based on its findings. If the company does not comply, the FDA may seek a court order authorizing the federal government to seize and destroy the product. FSIS likewise may request that a food product be recalled; to date, no such request has been refused. However, FSIS does have legal authority to seize and destroy meat and poultry products if they are thought to pose a serious hazard to public health. See FDA, "Food and Drug Administration Recall Policies," available at http://vm.cfsan.fda.gov/~lrd/recall2.html, and FSIS, "Food Recalls," available at http://www.fsis.usda.gov/OA/pubs/recallfocus.htm

points.[45] The HACCP rule represents a shift in FSIS's regulatory approach to include the production process as well as the finished product;[46] implementation of the HACCP system was completed in 2000.

The USDA has also worked in conjunction with the Department of Health and Human Services (HHS) in relation to food safety. In 1997, the two departments inaugurated a combined drive to enhance surveillance, risk assessment, research, inspection, and response to outbreaks.[47] This initiative expanded existing surveillance efforts, most notably FoodNet, and created the PulseNet program for molecular subtyping of foodborne bacteria. See the Appendix for further details.

Antimicrobial Drug Resistance

In 1999, HHS joined other federal agencies to form the Interagency Task Force on Antimicrobial Resistance, cochaired by representatives from the CDC, FDA, and NIH. This body recommended specific, coordinated federal actions to address the emerging threat of antimicrobial drug resistance through surveillance, prevention and control, research, and product development.[48] Some of the initiatives based on the agenda that the task force coordinates focus on developing systems to monitor antimicrobial drug use, educating physicians and the public about proper use of antibiotics, expanding

---

[45]FDA, "HAACP: A State-of-the-Art Approach to Food Safety," August 1999, available at http://vm.cfsan.fda.gov/~lrd/bghaccp.html, accessed July 26, 2001.

[46]USDA/FSIS, "Protecting the Public from Foodborne Illness: The Food Safety Inspection Service," April 2001, available at http://www.fsis.usda.gov/oa/background/fsisgeneral.htm, accessed July 24, 2001.

[47]FDA, USDA, U.S. Environmental Protection Agency, and CDC, "Food Safety from Farm to Table: A National Food Safety Initiative," report to the President, May 1997, available at http://www.cdc.gov/ncidod/foodsafe/report.htm, accessed August 3, 2001.

[48]Other members of the task force are HHS's Agency for Healthcare Research and Quality, the Health Care Financing Administration, the Health Resources and Services Administration, USDA, DoD, Department of Veterans Affairs, Environmental Protection Agency, and the U.S. Agency for International Development (USAID).

research of antimicrobial drug resistance, and facilitating development of new antimicrobial products.[49]

The food supply also has been recognized as a major source for the transmission of antimicrobial drug resistance from animals to humans.[50] To deal with this the National Antimicrobial Resistance Monitoring System (NARMS) for Enteric Bacteria has been set up to track susceptibility to 17 antimicrobial agents in humans and food animals and to yield information on trends that is used in developing regulations for the use of drugs in food and animal production.[51]

Biodefense Resources for Countering Infectious Disease

The threat of bioterrorism has spawned a number of initiatives and programs with "dual use" capabilities applicable to countering infectious diseases. Responsibility for managing public health and emergency medical preparedness for bioterrorism belongs primarily to the CDC and HHS's Office of Emergency Preparedness (OEP), although it is unclear how the new Office of Homeland Security will affect this arrangement. Some biodefense programs, particularly the National Pharmaceutical Stockpile (NPS) and National Disaster Medical System (NDMS), as well as some DoD assets have clear utility for mitigating catastrophic infectious disease epidemics.[52]

As part of the 1999 HHS bioterrorism initiative, the CDC was designated to lead the effort to improve the nation's public health capacity to respond to bioterrorism. The CDC's Bioterrorism Preparedness and Response Program oversees grant programs designed to

---

[49]HHS, "Antimicrobial Resistance: The Public Health Response," fact sheet, available at http://www.hhs.gov/news/press/2001pres/01fsdrugresistance.html, accessed June 28, 2001.

[50]Up to 35 percent of antibiotics produced in the United States are used in agriculture as feed supplements. Stuart Levy, American Society for Microbiology, "Antibiotic Resistance: Microbes on the Defense," in *Congressional Briefing: Infectious Diseases as We Enter the New Century: What Can We Do?* June 21, 1999, p. 5.

[51]CDC, "What Is NARMS?" available at http://www.cdc.gov/ncidod/dbmd/narms/what_is.htm, accessed August 16, 2001.

[52]"From 1997 to 2000, federal spending to prepare for [weapons of mass destruction] terrorism swelled from $130 million to $1.4 billion, a tenfold increase." Koblentz, "Overview of Federal Programs to Enhance State and Local Preparedness for Terrorism with Weapons of Mass Destruction," p. 3.

enhance state and local preparedness, epidemiology, and surveillance capabilities. Forty-two percent of the CDC's bioterrorism budget is devoted to enhancing state and local laboratory capabilities and communication.[53]

The CDC has delegated the management of the NPS to the Department of Veterans Affairs. This stockpile includes a range of pharmaceuticals and equipment for treating victims of a chemical or biological attack.[54] Eight immediate "push packages" are positioned in secure warehouses across the country, ready for deployment to the affected area within 12 hours of the federal decision to release NPS assets.[55] Technical Advisory Response Units, including pharmacists, public health experts, and emergency responders, will accompany the deployment of supplies to expedite transfer to local officials.[56] If additional medications are required, follow-up vendor-managed inventory supplies or packages, which are tailored to the situation, will arrive within 24 to 36 hours.[57]

The Federal Emergency Management Agency (FEMA) coordinates delivery of federal assistance to state and local governments in the event of a major emergency or disaster through the Federal Response Plan (FRP), a signed agreement among 27 federal departments and agencies.[58] The OEP in HHS is designated the lead agency for health

---

[53]Ibid., p. 1.

[54]These supplies include antibiotics (including those for the treatment and prophylaxis of anthrax, plague, and tularemia), chemical antidotes, antitoxins, life-support medications, intravenous administration and airway maintenance supplies, and medical and surgical items that would be used to supplement and resupply state and local public health agencies in the event of a biological or chemical terrorism incident.

[55]James M. Hughes, M.D., Director, National Center for Infectious Diseases, CDC, HHS, testimony before the Subcommittee on National Security, Veterans Affairs and International Relations, Committee on Government Reform, U.S. House of Representatives, May 1, 2001, available at http://www.hhs.gov.asl/testify/t010501a.html, accessed July 9, 2001.

[56]Ibid.

[57]CDC, "NPS Synopsis," available at http://www.cdc.gov/nceh/nps/synopses.htm, accessed July 6, 2001. It should be noted, however, that based on only a few recent cases of anthrax, the President asked for additional stockpiles of antibiotics. It is not clear that estimated requirements were made on reliable analyses of needed pharmaceuticals.

[58]Federal Emergency Management Agency, "FRP . . . at a Glance," available at http://www.fema.gov/r-n-r/frp/frpglnc.htm, accessed July 10, 2001.

and medical services within the FRP. The OEP manages the NDMS, an asset-sharing partnership among federal, state, and local governments; private industry; and civilian volunteers to provide medical assistance nationwide within 12 hours for up to 100,000 victims.[59]

In 1997, OEP established four National Medical Response Teams (NMRTs) designed to respond to incidents involving weapons of mass destruction. NMRTs have disease detection, decontamination, and medical care capabilities. Three of these teams may be deployed nationwide, while the fourth is stationed in Washington, D.C. Each NMRT has a standard supply of pharmaceuticals designed to treat 5,000 people exposed to chemical weapons and hundreds of people exposed to a biological agent. An additional stockpile may be loaned to localities or predeployed for special events.[60]

DoD has also developed programs to deal with bioterrorism. Two important initiatives are the Chemical and Biological Rapid Response Team (CB-RRT) and the Chemical and Biological Incident Response Force (CBIRF). Both of these bodies are able to provide additional detection, mitigation, decontamination, treatment, and remediation capabilities within four hours of the recognition of a chemical or biological event.[61]

Research

The search for diagnostic, therapeutic, and preventative measures to combat infectious disease depends on basic and applied biomedical research. As the nation's foremost institution in this area and with a budget of $23 billion, NIH is the major source of funding for U.S. research into infectious disease.[62] Within NIH, NIAID is the main

---

[59]HHS, "Office of Emergency Preparedness," available at http://www.oep.dhhs.gov/, accessed July 6, 2001.

[60]Koblentz, "Overview of Federal Programs to Enhance State and Local Preparedness for Terrorism with Weapons of Mass Destruction," pp. 33–34. OEP also manages the Metropolitan Medical Response System program for support of municipal emergency response to weapons of mass destruction events.

[61]Koblentz, p. 31; U.S. Army Technical Escort Unit, Web page, available at http://teu. sbccom.army.mil/index.htm, accessed September 6, 2001.

[62]Approximately 84 percent of the NIH budget supports extramural research conducted by more than 50,000 researchers at some 2,000 universities, hospitals, and

body charged with supporting studies to better understand, treat, and prevent infectious disease. NIAID sponsors and conducts research related to ecological and environmental factors influencing disease emergence, microbial changes and adaptations, human susceptibility to new microbes, and new and improved control strategies.[63] Four major areas are emphasized in this effort: global health and infectious diseases; HIV/AIDS; immune-mediated diseases such as allergy and asthma; and vaccines.[64] Basic research is typically directed toward development of vaccines, diagnostics, and drugs. However, NIAID has also funded projects aimed at sequencing the genomes of more than 50 pathogens, at least a dozen of which have already been mapped (including the bacteria that cause TB, gonorrhea, and cholera and the individual chromosomes of the malaria parasite, *P. falciparum*).[65]

DoD is also engaged in a variety of research areas that have applications for infectious disease detection, diagnosis, treatment, and prevention and defense. The U.S. Army Medical Research and Materiel Command (USAMRMC) is DoD's executive agent for medical chemical and biological defense (and combat) as well as telemedicine and infectious disease research. USAMRMC's Infectious Disease Program focuses on several areas, all of which have applications to the civilian world. These include the following:

- "Development of vaccines against militarily important diseases

- Discovery and development of prophylactic and treatment drugs for parasitic infectious diseases

- Techniques for rapid identification of disease organisms and diagnosis of infections

---

other research facilities. Eleven percent of the budget supports intramural research at NIH. HHS, "FY 2002 President's Budget for HHS," pp. 39–41.

[63]NIAID, "Infectious Diseases Research," available at http://www.niaid.nih.gov/eidr/mceid.htm, accessed July 5, 2001.

[64]Anthony S. Fauci, Director, NIAID, statement before the Subcommittee on Labor, Health, and Human Services and Education, U.S. House of Representatives, May 16, 2001, available at http://www.niaid.nih.gov/director/congress/2001/051601.htm, accessed August 28, 2001. See NIAID, "NIAID: Planning for the 21st Century," 2000, available at http://www.niaid.nih.gov/strategicplan2000/default.htm.

[65]Anthony S. Fauci, statement before the Subcommittee on Labor, Health and Human Services, and Education.

- Collection and analysis of epidemiological data that aid in the control of relevant infectious diseases

- Studies of control measures against infectious disease vectors."[66]

Global Surveillance and Response

Several federal agencies in the United States have been engaged in efforts to prevent and control infectious disease on a global scale. Many of those efforts have been initiated in coordination with other partners. These include foreign ministries of health, the WHO, the Pan American Health Organization, the UN Children's Fund (UNICEF), the World Bank, and others.

As the primary dispenser of foreign aid, USAID plays a major role in international efforts to counter infectious disease. Most efforts are aimed at building public health capacity in developing countries. USAID also leads the U.S. government response to the international HIV/AIDS crisis, having dedicated $1.6 billion toward prevention and control of the epidemic since 1986. In 2001, USAID distributed HIV/AIDS assistance to nongovernmental organizations in nearly 50 countries.[67] Other programs include an initiative to address antimicrobial resistance, TB, and malaria and a plan for surveillance and response through provision of technical assistance, applied research, and development of indigenous capacity.[68]

---

[66]This research has produced vaccines for hepatitis A and B, Japanese B encephalitis, Argentinian hemorrhagic fever, typhoid, adenovirus, and meningitis. U.S. Army Medical Research and Materiel Command, "RAD 1—Military Infectious Disease Research Program," available at http://mrmc-www.army.mil/, accessed October 15, 2001. An additional military initiative is the Unconventional Pathogen Countermeasures Program at the Defense Advanced Research Projects Agency (DARPA), which sponsors a number of projects that seek novel ways to detect and protect against pathogens. Another DoD program, DARPA's Advanced Diagnostics program, aims to develop "the capability to detect in the body—in real time and in the absence of recognizable signs and symptoms and when pathogen numbers are still low—the presence of infection by any pathogen."

[67]USAID, "USAID: Leading the Global Fight Against HIV/AIDS," available at http://www.usaid.gov/press/releases/2001/fs010420_4.html, accessed August 13, 2001.

[68]USAID, "Reducing the Threat of Infectious Diseases of Major Public Health Importance: USAID's Initiative to Prevent and Control Infectious Diseases," March 1998, p. 3, available at www.usaid.gov/pop_health/pdf/idfstrategy.pdf.

The CDC also plays a role in international health activities because all disease outbreaks have the potential to impact the United States. In fact, the CDC's support of international disease control and prevention is considered a key institutional objective. Much of this work is carried out through the CISET Emerging Infectious Disease Task Force.[69] Six priority areas for international cooperation have been identified: outbreak assistance, disease surveillance, applied research, dissemination of public health tools, support of global initiatives for disease control, and public health training and capacity building.[70]

The CDC is seen as a world leader in outbreak investigation. Epidemiologic Assistance (EPI-AIDs) is available to respond to foreign outbreaks (when requested); in FY 2000, EIS officers participated in 11 overseas investigations.[71] The CDC also collaborates with USAID, the WHO, and others on disease-specific surveillance and control efforts, particularly targeting HIV/AIDS, measles, TB, and malaria.[72]

Finally, DoD is playing an increasingly important role in global disease surveillance, particularly with regard to building epidemiological capacity of foreign laboratories. Apart from the GEIS initiative noted above, DoD has established an HIV/AIDS Prevention Program, which is run by the Naval Health Research Center as a component of

---

[69]CDC, "Preventing Emerging Infectious Diseases," p. 47.

[70]From CDC's soon-to-be-released global strategy, Protecting Our Nation's Health in an Era of Globalization: CDC's Global Infectious Disease Strategy, forthcoming. See also Bruce Brown et al., "Setting Priorities for Global Infectious Disease Control," *U.S Medicine*, April 2001, available at http://www.usmedicine.com/column.cfm?column ID=44&issueID=25, accessed July 6, 2001.

[71]CDC, "Requests for Epidemiologic Assistance (EPI-AIDs)."

[72]The CDC has been designated as the lead agency within HHS to implement the Leadership and Investment for Fighting an Epidemic Initiative, addressing HIV/AIDS in India and Africa. To foster more local capacity, the CDC has established 25 Field Epidemiology Training Programs around the world. These training programs, modeled on the EIS, have graduated more than 1,200 participants since 1980. In addition, the CDC supports research centers in Botswana, Cote d'Ivoire, Guatemala, Kenya, and Thailand and houses more than 40 WHO Collaborating Centers in the United States, each addressing a specific global health problem. CDC and Agency for Toxic Substances Disease Registry (ATSDR), "Working with Partners to Improve Global Health: A Strategy for CDC and ATSDR," September 2000, p. 4, available at http://www. cdc.gov/ogh/pub/execsummary.pdf, and CDC, "International Training Programs for Applied Epidemiology and Global Health Leadership," available at http://www.cdc. gov/programs/global5.htm, accessed August 15, 2001.

the U.S. participation in the International Partnership Against HIV/AIDS in Africa. The program received $10 million in 2000 to establish training and prevention programs aimed at reducing the spread of HIV among military personnel in select African countries. The long-term aim is to integrate the prevention activities of USAID, CDC, and the Health Resources and Services Administration for application to African military communities.[73]

ASSESSMENT OF U.S. CAPABILITIES TO COUNTER INFECTIOUS DISEASES

While the various initiatives described above have helped to provide the United States with one of the most advanced public health systems in the world, several critical weaknesses are currently serving to undermine the effectiveness of U.S. disease prevention and mitigation efforts. Principal areas of concern include the inadequacy of surveillance mechanisms; fiscal neglect; a lack of personnel, especially those with experience in recognizing and treating emerging infections; a shrinking capacity to produce needed vaccines and therapeutics; and a lack of coordination for many of these functions.

Surveillance

Surveillance is key to the prevention of epidemics. However, adequate monitoring capabilities do not exist uniformly across the United States. As Davis and Lederberg note, "Although a tremendous amount of surveillance is accomplished [in the United States], much of it is disease-specific, resulting in disjointed programs and

---

[73]Naval Health Research Center, "DoD HIV/AIDS Prevention Program," available at http://www.nhrc.navy.mil/programs/life/managementplan.html, accessed August 30, 2001. It should be noted that the International Services branch of the USDA's Animal and Plant Health Inspection Service (IS/APHIS), which seeks to safeguard U.S. agriculture from foreign pests and diseases, additionally plays a role in overseas disease monitoring. Operating in 27 countries, IS/APHIS works to ensure that foreign agricultural officials understand and adhere to U.S. agricultural health policies and import regulations. For further details, see APHIS, "International Services," available at http://www.aphis.usda.gov/is/, accessed August 17, 2001.

unsustainable systems supported by categorical funding."[74] Increased trade, travel, changes in agricultural practice, and other factors further exacerbate difficulties in surveillance, heightening problems associated with performing effective epidemiological investigations.[75]

A lack of adequate surveillance mechanisms not only compounds the problem of correctly identifying and assessing appropriate control-and-prevention tools. It also makes it more difficult to recognize new diseases, discriminate among geographically separated but epidemiologically linked outbreaks, detect factors responsible for illnesses, and identify a potential bioterrorist attack.

Indicative of this was a 1999 General Accounting Office (GAO) review of U.S. infectious-disease surveillance capabilities, which concluded that laboratory capabilities vary from state to state and are not comprehensive with most jurisdictions surveying only five of six important diseases and many ignoring hepatitis C and penicillin-resistant *S. pneumoniae*.[76] The unavoidable message of the GAO assessment was that the U.S. first line of defense against diseases is severely impeded and requires considerable investment in the development of significantly improved and coordinated surveillance capabilities.

Fiscal Neglect

Surveillance is only one part of the larger public health infrastructure, and it has been recognized in many studies that America's overall system has worsened significantly over the last quarter century due to fiscal neglect.[77] According to the Health Care Financing

---

[74]Jonathan R. Davis and Joshua Lederberg, eds., *Public Health Systems and Emerging Infections: Assessing the Capabilities of the Public and Private Sectors—Workshop Summary*, Washington, D.C.: National Academy Press, 2001, p. 6.

[75]Ibid. p. 1.

[76]As cited in Davis and Lederberg, p. 90. See also GAO, "Emerging Infectious Diseases: Consensus on Needed Laboratory Capacity Could Strengthen Surveillance," 1999.

[77]For instance, U.S. Senate, "Bioterrorism: Public Health and Medical Preparedness," statement by Janet Heinrich, October 9, 2001, before the Senate Subcommittee on Public Health, GAO-02-141T; and Advisory Panel to Assess Domestic Response Capabilities for Terrorism Involving Weapons of Mass Destruction, *Second Annual Report to the President and the Congress—II: Toward a National Strategy for Combating Terrorism*, Santa Monica, Calif.: RAND, December 15, 2000.

Administration (HCFA), only 3 percent of the $1.1 trillion the United States spent on healthcare was devoted to explicit public health activities. Slightly more than 50 percent of U.S. expenditures were dedicated to hospital care and physician services, while drugs and other nonmedical durables accounted for 11 percent of the budget.[78]

As a result of insufficient financial resources, laboratories crucial to the identification of diseases have become increasingly ill-equipped to deal with outbreaks when they occur. This has not only affected diagnostic capabilities at the state level (the current effectiveness of which varies greatly from one region to the next), it has also detracted from appropriate capacity federally.[79]

A lack of resources has also at least partly detracted from the development of a modern information-sharing system that is able to overcome historical difficulties in communicating across state lines; among federal, state, and local officials; and among emergency rooms, hospitals, and government departments. The anthrax attacks in fall 2001 exemplify the difficulties currently facing the United States in this regard. Although public health authorities in Washington, D.C., were aware of cases that had arisen in Florida, and the presence of anthrax spores in the Senate offices had been disclosed in a timely manner, physicians in the nation's capital were not alerted. As a result, at least two postal workers exposed to the agent were identified only after it was too late for effective treatment.[80] If more individuals had been affected or if there had been no advance

---

[78]National Health Care Anti-Fraud Association, "Impact of Fraud: U.S. Healthcare Spending," fact sheets, available at http://www.nhcaa.org/factsheet_impact.htm, accessed December 15, 2001.

[79]GAO, "West Nile Virus Outbreak," pp. 26–32. Indicative of this is that there is just a single full-time employee dedicated to the CDC's reference laboratory for plague (the only one in the world). As a direct result of this paucity of experience and knowledge, two of the five people in the United States who contracted plague in 1996 died of the disease before it was even identified. See "Fatal Human Plague—Arizona and Colorado, 1996," MMWR, Vol. 46, No. 27, July 11, 1997, pp. 617–620.

[80]"Update: Investigation of Bioterrorism-Related Anthrax and Interim Guidelines for Exposure Management and Antimicrobial Therapy, October 2001," MMWR, Vol. 50, No. 42, October 26, 2001, pp. 910–919, available at http://www.cdc.gov/mmwr/preview/mmwrhtml/mm5042a1.htm, accessed June 22, 2002; Elizabeth Becker and Robin Toner, "A Nation Challenged: The Victims, Postal Workers' Illness Set Off No Alarms," New York Times, October 24, 2001, p. B1.

warning, the overall seriousness of the crisis would likely have been far worse.

Personnel

Insufficient staffing at all levels and in all sectors of the medical and public health communities is emerging as a significant threat in the United States, not least because an adequate number of educated and trained personnel is critical to maintaining necessary public health and medical capabilities. The GAO has cited a lack of laboratory personnel as one of the primary problems facing laboratories today, largely because it detracts from state and local laboratory capabilities to perform infectious disease surveillance.[81] Nurses are also in critically short supply, and this problem is expected to worsen. By 2020, based on current trends in supply and requirements, there is expected to be a 20 percent deficit in the overall nurse workforce, which will mean that other, less-trained individuals will have to take over nursing duties, potentially putting patients at severe risk.[82]

Shortages of nurses and other staff are already emerging as a significant problem. During the 1999–2000 flu season, demand exceeded hospital capabilities across the country, affecting the ability to provide definitive treatment to those suffering from the virus as well as those concurrently in need of other types of care.[83] Assessing the situation, Mary Beachley, president of the Maryland Nurses Association, stated, "If a major super bug hit, we'd be in trouble. Our response in the short-term would be okay, but long-term care with large numbers of critically ill patients [would] be a problem."[84]

---

[81]Janet Heinrich, "Health Workforce: Ensuring Adequate Supply and Distribution Remains Challenging," Washington, D.C.: GAO, August 1, 2001.

[82]P. Buerhaus, D. Staiger, and D. Auerbach, "Implications of an Aging Registered Nurse Workforce," *JAMA*, Vol. 283, No. 22, June 14, 2000, pp. 2948–2954. A number of studies have found that healthcare quality is related to the nursing staff's education level and the number of registered nurses on staff.

[83]M. Schoch-Spana, "Hospitals Buckle During Normal Flu Season: Implications for Bioterrorism Response," *Biodefense Quarterly*, Vol. 1, No. 4, March 2000, available at http://www.hopkins-biodefense.org/pages/news/quarter1_4.html, accessed December 15, 2001.

[84]As quoted in Schoch-Spana.

Lack of Experience with Exotic Infectious Diseases

In addition to the sheer lack of bodies, many doctors and other healthcare workers lack the knowledge and experience to recognize uncommon infectious diseases. Because these personnel are often the first line of defense in diagnosing and containing outbreaks, this deficiency in expertise can be highly deleterious. Again, the 2001 anthrax attacks provide a pertinent case in point. The New York Public Health Laboratory dismissed the initial diagnosis of cutaneous anthrax ascribed to Erin O'Connor, the National Broadcasting Company (NBC) employee who was one of the first to exhibit symptoms of the disease, because no spores were detected in her tissue samples. It was not until Robert Stevens contracted inhalation anthrax and Ms. O'Connor went to an infectious disease specialist that she was confirmed to have skin anthrax. The doctor who made the correct diagnosis had experience in developing countries, enabling him to recognize the characteristic anthrax lesion.[85]

Shrinking Vaccine Production Capacity

One of the most effective tools in improving the U.S. ability to deal with infectious disease has been the widespread use of vaccines (especially in children), which played a large role in reducing polio, measles, mumps, rubella, chicken pox, and other serious diseases.

These gains are at risk for a number of reasons. First, because many infectious diseases are unknown in North America today, people are less willing to chance the rare adverse reaction to vaccines. Perceived risks have been further magnified by those who have legitimate, though not necessarily science-based, concerns about immunization safety as well as the political controversy surrounding the mandated anthrax vaccine program in the U.S. military (which was in place from May 1998 through early 2000). Second, funding for public health initiatives has declined substantially, and many vaccines no longer enjoy the financial support from states that they once did. Finally, the vaccine industry has become progressively more concentrated, with only four major pharmaceutical firms currently

---

[85]Lawrence K. Altman, "A Nation Challenged: NBC; Doctor in City Reported Anthrax Case Before Florida," *New York Times,* October 18, 2001, p. B7.

engaging in production: Merck, Aventis-Pasteur, Glaxo, and Wyeth-Ayerst (although several smaller biotech companies are also involved in vaccine development). Many critical vaccines are also made by only one FDA-approved supplier, which has put the United States at great risk of losing an already limited manufacturing capability. Problems have already been encountered with the production of influenza, tetanus, diphtheria toxoid, and adenovirus vaccines.[86]

The time to develop new vaccines is long, and the cost is high: 10 to 15 years and $300 million to $500 million.[87] Given this reality, it is highly unlikely the United States will be able to quickly ramp up its vaccine production. This puts Americans at risk and means immigrants settling in the country may not be able to acquire immunity, which obviously places other susceptible individuals at risk.[88, 89]

Insufficient Attention to the Provision of Global Healthcare Aid

While the United States has been engaged in various international efforts to prevent and control infectious disease, it has been relatively inactive in terms of global healthcare aid. Vaccine research and

[86]Prior to February 2001, Aventis-Pasteur and Wyeth-Ayerst Laboratories produced tetanus and diphtheria toxoid, but Wyeth ceased production without warning. Although Aventis ramped up production, because the vaccine takes 11 months to produce, a shortage was created in the short term. "Notice to Readers: Deferral of Routine Booster Doses of Tetanus and Diphtheria Toxoids for Adolescents and Adults," *MMWR*, Vol. 50, No. 20, May 25, 2001, pp. 418, 427.

[87]According to one estimate by Pharmaceutical Research and Manufacturers of America, drug companies spend an average of 12 to 15 years to develop a new drug at an average cost of $500 million, http://www.phrma.org/publications/documents/factsheets/2001-03-01.210.phtml, accessed November 30, 2001.

[88]The Immigration and Naturalization Service has in fact currently waived the requirement for tetanus-diphtheria vaccination for immigrants due to the shortage in supply. See http://www.cdc.gov/ncidod/dq/technica.htm, accessed November 30, 2001; the deferral is in effect until March 31, 2002.

[89]For additional information on vaccine production challenges, see "Vaccines Research, Development, Production and Procurement Issues," in *Biological Threats and Terrorism: Assessing the Science and Response Capabilities*, Knobler, S. L., A. A. F. Mahmoud, and L. A. Pray, eds., Forum on Emerging Infections, Board on Global Health, 2002, pp. 85–121; *Calling the Shots*, Committee on Immunization Finance Policies and Practices, Division of Health Care Services and Division of Health Promotion and Disease Prevention, Institute of Medicine, National Academy Press, Washington, D.C., 2000.

development has tended to focus on viral strains prevalent in North America as opposed to Africa and Asia—precisely the areas where disease threat is most widespread—and has only recently and hesitantly begun to embrace the idea of subsidizing to ensure lower guaranteed dosage prices. Also, comparatively few resources have been made available to help poor countries boost the effectiveness of their overall public medical systems and address some of the conditions contributing to the emergence and spread of pathogenic agents within their borders.[90] Indeed, health issues have consistently failed to figure prominently in Washington's external aid priorities, the delineation of which has tended to be governed by a more reality-grounded focus on political concerns.

According to the World Bank's Commission on Macroeconomics and Health, $27 billion, which equates to just 0.1 percent of the collective GDP of the United States, Japan, and Europe, would be sufficient to ensure that cheap, tried-and-tested treatments, such as vaccines and gastrointestinal oral rehydration therapy, were made widely available throughout much of the developing world.[91] Certainly the United States should not be expected to shoulder the entire burden of this fiscal effort. The chief responsibility for fighting disease in poor states must, ultimately, lie with the governments of these countries. This being said, it is an area where Washington is better placed than most to play a meaningful role—particularly in light of the fact that it took Congress only three days following the September 11 attacks in New York and Washington to appropriate $40 billion for the war against global terrorism.[92] Moreover, the exercise of such leadership would create an opportunity to demonstrate an appealing style of benign American hegemony, whereby the United States could be seen (and recognized) as willing to articulate and act on shared interests rather than simple, narrowly defined, national priorities.[93]

---

[90]See, for instance, CSIS, *Contagion and Conflict*, pp. 54–55, and "Terrorism Is Not the Only Scourge," *The Economist*, December 22, 2001.

[91]World Bank, "Macroeconomics and Health: Investing in Health for Economic Development," report of the World Bank Commission on Macroeconomics and Health, December 2001, available at http://www.cmhealth.org/index.html. See also World Bank Commission on Macroeconomics and Health, cited in "The Health of Nations," *The Economist*, December 22, 2001.

[92]"Terrorism Is Not the Only Scourge," *The Economist*.

[93]CSIS, *Contagion and Conflict*, p. 63.

Lack of Coordination

The lack of clear leadership, coordination, and communication in the area of infectious disease clearly poses a threat to the United States. Within the federal government, numerous agencies and centers, including the CDC, FDA, NIH, DoD, USAID, USDA, U.S. Fish and Wildlife Services, and the Department of the Interior, work on various aspects of preparation and response. In addition, because public health is a state function, numerous agencies and mechanisms exist at the subfederal level. Add to this the responsibilities of the private sector and a highly complex patchwork arrangement emerges to deal with everything from prevention to surveillance to treatment and containment.

A lack of communication has frequently resulted in the delayed recognition of new or unusual diseases, as the 2001 anthrax cases illustrate. This problem has been compounded by the fact that hospitals often do not share adequate information with the local health department, generally waiting for laboratory- or specialist-based diagnoses before reporting incidents to the relevant authorities.[94]

Because infectious disease represents a ubiquitous, wide-ranging threat to the security of the United States, it is essential that this particular manifestation of the GAP challenge be dealt with in a coordinated and systematic manner. While some functions are clearly best performed at the local and state levels, standards and resources must flow from the federal government to ensure uniform protection of America and its citizens. Given the rapidity with which viral and bacterial agents spread and emerge or reemerge, it is critical that Washington move quickly to better integrate and augment the overall disease mitigation system at its disposal. The final chapter presents some initial policy recommendations for achieving such an outcome.

---

[94]George Washington University, "Preparing for a Bioterrorist Incident: Linking the Public Health and Medical Communities," National Health Policy Forum, October 4–5, 1999, site visit to Baltimore and Fort Detrick, Maryland.

Chapter Six

CONCLUSION

This report has highlighted infectious disease as a serious risk both to the international system and to the United States. The overall threat is being driven by globalization, inadvertent consequences stemming from modern medical and agricultural practices, behavioral changes, environmental factors such as climatic change, and the growing danger of bioterrorism. The study specifically recognizes that microbial challenges cannot be territorially bounded and, therefore, need to be understood and dealt with in a larger global context. Further, the analysis delineates disease as a highly pervasive influence that not only impinges on security in terms of traditional conceptions of state stability, but, more insidiously, directly undermines and weakens the essential socioeconomic foundations upon which any effective polity ultimately depends.

The urgency of the infectious disease challenge currently confronting the global community cannot be ignored. People in both the developed and the developing worlds are being exposed on a daily basis to new and reemerging pathogens, a pattern that is continually exacerbated by factors as wide-ranging as globalization, the use and misuse of medical and agricultural technological advances, unsustainable urbanization, environmental degradation, and changing social and behavioral patterns.

The impact of HIV/AIDS in South Africa exemplifies the extreme challenges that a country and its citizens can face at all levels when a deadly disease afflicts a large portion of the populace. The behavior of both individuals and the society as a whole—such as the prevalence of unprotected sex, the poor treatment of women, and the lack of a proactive response by the government—has exacerbated the spread of HIV as well as amplified its consequences, in terms of human life, confidence in government, political stability, and world standing. The HIV/AIDS epidemic has, in fact, left South Africa unprepared to meet its external military and, arguably, internal security obligations; incapable of fully meeting its economic potential; and ill-equipped to provide for the most basic social and health needs of its citizens.

The United States has a myriad of programs and processes for combating the threat of infectious disease, most of which rest in local and state hands. While the CDC provides a level of integration for these assets and federal dollars have been set aside to help improve their effectiveness, overall national coordination and management remain ad hoc and disparate. Just as important, authority and resources vary widely across jurisdictions, at both the federal and the state and local levels. The result has been an underfunded and poorly coordinated public health infrastructure that is currently serving to impede U.S. disease surveillance, prevention, and response efforts.

Further compounding the situation is the fact that the provision of U.S. foreign aid is largely based on narrow political, rather than more comprehensive health security, concerns. This has diverted scarce resources away from the areas where they are needed most and, in so doing, left many regions of the world as potential reservoirs of disease input into the country.

To be sure, the September 11, 2001, attacks on the World Trade Center and the Pentagon, combined with the heightened fear of bioterrorism stemming from the 2001 anthrax crisis, have focused attention on the need for a strong public health infrastructure, and policymakers have begun to make funds available to address some of the fundamental shortcomings inherent in the system. However, this investment must be sustained and there is considerable work to do in enhancing overall policy coordination, management, and development.

The federal government should consider playing a more concerted role in providing resources and instituting unified standards to provide consistent microbial protection across the country. At the same time, however, the nature of infectious diseases necessarily means that state and local authorities need to retain a measure of flexibility in implementing programs and ensuring that they are best able to meet their needs. Moreover, as noted in Chapter Five, public health issues remain a state function in the U.S. system, statutory authority for which, therefore, cannot constitutionally rest solely in federal hands.

Within this general context, there are several specific and direct measures that could be instituted to address the shortcomings identified in this study:

- Coordination among public health authorities at all levels of government needs to be substantially enhanced and developed in conjunction with mechanisms that allow for greater interaction across state borders and local boundaries. Progress in this area should proceed in conjunction with moves both to better integrate stovepipe surveillance systems and data formats and to expand existing capabilities for detecting and identifying infectious diseases through extramural research in universities and other academic centers. Increased federal investment is critical to these endeavors and could provide the basis from which to develop a functional, coherent national policy for combating infectious disease.

- Greater thought needs to be given to how to involve the private sector in overall public health efforts, particularly in relation to the research, development, and manufacture of vaccines and antibiotics and the development of microbial surveillance technology. Options that the federal government might consider in this regard include funding basic research in appropriate areas and subsidizing the market for new products by agreeing to guarantee minimum purchasing contracts. The need for vaccines and appropriate medical devices to protect the military and civilian populations from biological agents should provide sufficient political justification to underwrite incentives of this sort.

- A large-scale education and information campaign should be undertaken to explain the need for regular vaccination and highlight the importance of disease prevention through such practices as protected sex, the responsible administration of antibiotics, and "clean" needle exchanges. These programs must be conceived in such a way that they are not overly scientific—i.e., that their meaning is not lost on the layperson (as has occurred in South Africa with the AIDS publicity drive). They must also be carefully managed to ensure that they raise awareness and understanding without unduly heightening public anxiety and fear.

- Efforts should be made to augment the supply of healthcare workers currently available in the country. One relatively quick way to achieve this would be to create a dedicated public health service reserve that can be activated in the case of an emergency. This supplemental force could be trained for relatively low-level medical and public health duties, such as administering drugs and vaccinations, and retained on a schedule similar to that of military reservists—one weekend a month and two weeks a year. Over the longer term, funds will need to be invested to ensure the sustained provision of personnel with more advanced skills and training. To this end, monies should be directed toward supporting public health educational components at universities as well as facilitating ongoing professional training, particularly in the areas of disease detection, identification, diagnosis, and treatment.

- Hospitals and emergency health facilities need to develop appropriate modalities for dealing with sudden crises and patient influxes, such as those that might occur in the aftermath of a bioterrorist attack. Medical receiving facilities should have the means to provide surge capacity in hospital beds and other vital functional areas and have in place auxiliary communication systems and power networks. Since regional or national transportation is likely to be affected by a terrorist event, hospitals should also have a plan to access backup laboratory facilities and procedures when they are unable to use their usual diagnostic services.

- More resources need to be invested in foreign governments to help them increase the effectiveness of their internal disease prevention efforts. Useful initiatives that could be undertaken include mutual aid agreements for the sharing of biological intelligence, research, diagnostics, personnel, vaccines, antibiotics, medical devices, and treatment/prevention techniques; help with the creation of dedicated regional health surveillance networks; assistance to promote sustainable urban development and regeneration schemes; and focused response efforts to deal with specific disease-promoting catalysts (such as unprotected sex and the spread of AIDS and other STDs in southern Africa).

Beyond these six health-oriented initiatives, the United States also needs to revisit how it defines security and formulates mechanisms for its provision. Institutional structures that have traditionally focused on narrow, statecentric concerns will have to be expanded and developed to accommodate challenges that threaten broader societal interests. Increased cooperation among agencies and departments that have historically had little to do with one another— including defense, justice, intelligence, public health, agriculture, and environment—will also be required, as will new executive functions to coordinate such multidimensional policy responses.[1]

One specific area calling for drastic change is the field of national intelligence. Bodies such as the CIA and Defense Intelligence Agency (DIA) will have to become familiar with new operational contexts that require different analytical techniques, skills, mandates, and information-handling methods. Threat assessments and forecasts will need to be more closely grounded on scientifically formulated models that integrate the work of the medical research sector on new and reemerging diseases. Just as important, security analysts will need to devote greater attention to the epidemiological literature as part of their regular reading "diet." Overseas monitoring activities will also need to encompass a somewhat wider ambit, focusing on such things as the effectiveness of national medical screening systems; prevailing geopolitical, social, economic, and environmental conditions that affect disease incidence; and state compliance with international health conventions and agreements. Indeed, countries that do not pose an obvious military security danger may be the ones most likely to pose a disease risk, owing to poorly developed and

---

[1]Plans to establish a Department of Homeland Security could provide a useful precedent and model in this regard. Although specifically directed to counter terrorism, the new department will represent the first institutionalization of an integrated, interdepartmental body that has both programmatic and budgetary powers within the U.S. security structure. See, for instance, "White House Sets Out Blueprint for Homeland Security," *Financial Times*, June 19, 2002.

underfunded public health systems. Such possibilities will need to be recognized and factored into strategic threat analyses.[2]

Given the influence that the United States retains in such major military/security-focused organizations as the North Atlantic Treaty Organization (NATO), Washington could, finally, play a leading role in adapting these institutions to take on a more specific public and global health role. New functional areas that might conceivably be instituted in this regard include disease crisis and consequence management through the provision of early warning and response indicators, backed up by ongoing and concerted global epidemiological surveillance.[3] In developing such mandates, the United States could usefully capitalize on the nascent multitask framework that has already been established for collective political-military humanitarian missions around the world.

Measures such as these will require ongoing political input and sustained financial commitment. Reform along the lines suggested above will require federal support as well as a better understanding of public health issues and how they affect national and global resilience and stability. Considerable policy attention and resources have already been devoted to shoring up defenses against the relatively low-probability scenario of a large-scale bioterrorist attack.[4] By contrast, modalities for dealing with naturally occurring microbes and pathogens, which every year inflict a significant and growing human and economic toll, remain relatively underdeveloped. Serious assessments of the threat posed by infectious diseases suggest that this imbalance needs to be modified, as a matter of both fiscal responsibility and judicious public policy.

---

[2]Simon Dalby has made many of these same arguments in relation to intelligence reform to deal with environmental threats to national security. See his "Security, Intelligence, the National Interest and the Global Environment."

[3]Recommendations of this sort were highlighted during a transnational issues session of the "Euro-Atlantic Relationship: Ready for the Global Era?" Wilton Park Conference, Wilton Park, UK, May 21–25, 2001.

[4]More than $3 billion has been requested to prevent, detect, and treat terror-related health threats in FY 2002. See Helen Dewar, "Senate Bioterrorism Bill Doubles Bush's Request," *Washington Post*, November 16, 2001, p. A15.

CDC SURVEILLANCE AND COLLECTION SYSTEMS

National Notifiable Disease Surveillance System (NNDSS) is a database maintained by the CDC's Epidemiology Program Office. NNDSS is a mechanism for the collection and publication of surveillance data gathered by state health departments on specific diseases and conditions. The system is based on a list of notifiable diseases compiled annually by the Council of State and Territorial Epidemiologists (CSTE) in collaboration with the CDC.[1]

National Electronic Disease Surveillance System (NEDSS) is a planned CDC disease surveillance network that will be developed from existing technology and data. It will be based on existing technology and will link critical healthcare facilities and components of the local emergency medical systems to public health agencies for ongoing pathogenic monitoring and reporting.[2]

Epidemiology and Laboratory Capacity (ELC) is a program that assists state and local health departments in developing capabilities to

---

[1]The CDC's list of "notifiable" diseases is published annually in *Morbidity and Mortality Weekly Report* (MMWR) as "Summary of Notifiable Diseases, United States." Each year the CSTE recommends additions to and deletions from this list. Roush et al., "Mandatory Reporting of Diseases and Conditions by Health Care Professionals and Laboratories," p. 164.

[2]U.S. Senate, statement by James Hughes made before the Subcommittee on Technology, Terrorism and Government Information Subcommittee on Youth Violence Committee on the Judiciary, April 20, 1999, and U.S. House of Representatives, statement made by Scott Lillibridge before the Subcommittee on National Security, Veterans Affairs and International Relations Committee on Government Reform, September 22, 1999.

- identify and monitor the occurrence of infectious diseases of public health importance in a community,

- characterize disease determinants,

- identify and respond to disease outbreaks and other infectious disease emergencies,

- use public health data for priority setting and policy development, and

- assess the effectiveness of their prevention-and-control activities.[3]

The **Emerging Infection Program (EIP)** aims to assess both the public health impact of emerging infections and the measures used to prevent and control them. Currently operating in nine states, the EIP network sponsors the Active Bacterial Core Surveillance Program and the Foodborne Disease Active Surveillance Network (FoodNet). EIP also provides funding to selected sites for electronic, laboratory-based surveillance and reporting of meningoencephalitis, chronic liver disease, and acute viral hepatitis and surveillance for the Unexplained Deaths and Critical Illnesses Due to Possibly Infectious Causes project, which seeks to identify and characterize emerging pathogens.

Enhanced Surveillance Project has been developed for syndromic surveillance at special events. Syndrome baseline data are established using emergency room visit data at sentinel hospitals. The CDC analyzes the data to detect aberrations and notifies the state and local health departments of problems requiring epidemiological investigation.[4]

---

[3]CDC, "Epidemiology and Laboratory Capacity (ELC) for Infectious Diseases Cooperative Agreement," available at http://www.cdc.gov/ncidod/osr/ELC.htm, accessed July 11, 2001.

[4]CDC, "Enhanced Surveillance Project (ESP)," available at http://www.bt.cdc.gov/EpiSurv/ESP.asp, accessed August 8, 2001. This system has been used at special events, including the Democratic and Republican national conventions, the World Trade Organization meeting in Seattle, and the Super Bowl in Tampa, Florida.

Four provider-based sentinel networks have been established to monitor conditions not covered by routine health department surveillance:

- *Emergency Department Sentinel Network for Emerging Infections* is a network of 11 university-affiliated, urban hospital emergency departments for responding to new diseases or epidemics. The network currently investigates *Shiga* toxin-producing *E. coli*, rabies postexposure prophylaxis practices, and nosocomial *M. tuberculosis* transmission in emergency departments. The network plans to add studies of antimicrobial use, meningitis, and encephalitis to its agenda.[5]

- *Infectious Diseases Society of America, Emerging Infections Network* (IDSA EIN), a sentinel network of more than 700 physicians specializing in infectious diseases, grew out of a 1995 CDC Cooperative Agreement Program award to the Infectious Diseases Society of America. EIN is designed to function as an "early warning system" for the CDC by supplying information about unusual cases encountered by the network's members.[6]   Network physicians also agree to assist the public health community by supplying information on diagnostic and therapeutic approaches to specific syndromes and infections and preliminary estimates on morbidity and mortality.[7]

- *GeoSentinel* was first funded by the CDC's Division of Quarantine in 1996 and consists of 25 travel/tropical medicine clinics around

---

[5]CDC, "Surveillance Systems Home Pages and Contacts," available at http://www.cdc.gov/ncidod/osr/survsyss.htm#EMERGE, accessed July 3, 2001.

[6]Infectious Disease Society of America, "Emerging Infections Network," available at http://www.idsociety.org/EIN/TOC.htm, accessed July 11, 2001.

[7]Every six to eight weeks EIN members receive two-page requests for information about specific clinical entities. Members may also submit spontaneous reports. In the event of a possible outbreak, EIN members may receive e-mail or facsimile requests for information, to which they are expected to respond within 24 hours. Summaries of information collected by periodic queries, urgent queries, and spontaneous reports are sent to all EIN members, the CDC, and state and territorial epidemiologists. Infectious Disease Society of America, "Emerging Infections Network: Background and Organization," www.idsociety.org/EIN/AboutEIN.htm, accessed July 27, 2001.

the world that monitor geographic and temporal trends in morbidity among travelers and other globally mobile populations.[8]

- *Border Infectious Disease Surveillance (BIDS)* is a binational disease surveillance project that conducts active sentinel surveillance for hepatitis and febrile-rash illnesses, such as measles and dengue, at nine sites on the U.S.-Mexican border. The BIDS project represents collaboration among the CDC, U.S. and Mexican state health departments, the Mexican Secretariat of Health, and the Pan American Health Organization.[9]

Global Emerging Infections Surveillance and Response System (GEIS) is a network of domestic and overseas military research units charged with supporting global surveillance, training, research, and response to infectious disease.[10] Five Army and Navy laboratories in Egypt, Kenya, Indonesia, Peru, and Thailand monitor infectious diseases of concern to the military and host countries, particularly influenza, drug-resistant malaria, and diarrheal and febrile diseases. Through close working relationships with host country counterparts, DoD-GEIS personnel have also served to improve local epidemiolog-

---

[8]CDC, "Surveillance Systems Home Pages and Contacts." The network's basic surveillance tool is a one-page faxable form submitted by participating clinics to a central data site. Diagnoses may be entered as specific etiologies or as syndromes. GeoSentinel also has the capability to request urgent surveys of all 25 sites; send inquiries to 350 medical providers via TravelMed, the international Society of Travel Medicine list service; and electronically disseminate alerts to 1,250 society's providers in 65 countries. International Society of Travel Medicine, "GeoSentinel: Objectives," available at http://www.istm.org/geosweb/objectiv.html, accessed August 7, 2001.

[9]Surveillance is conducted at San Diego, California/Tijuana; Baja California; Nogales, Arizona; Nogales, Sonora; Las Cruces, New Mexico/El Paso, Texas/Ciudad Juarez, Chihuahua; and McAllen, Texas/Reynosa, Tamaulipas. CDC, "Border Infectious Disease Surveillance Project Moves Forward," *NCID Focus*, Vol. 1, No. 2, March–April 2000, p. 4; CDC, "Surveillance Resources: Surveillance Systems," available at http://www.cdc.ncidod/osr/survsyss.htm, accessed July 3, 2001.

[10]Domestic components of DoD-GEIS are the U.S. Army Center for Health Promotion and Preventive Medicine, Aberdeen Proving Ground, Maryland; USAMRIID, Fort Detrick, Maryland; the Naval Health Research Center, San Diego, California; the Naval Environmental Health Center, Norfolk, Virginia; and the U.S. Air Force Global Surveillance Office, Brooks AFB, Texas. The GEIS overseas laboratories are the Armed Forces Research Institute of Medical Sciences, Bangkok, Thailand; the U.S. Army Medical Research Unit, Nairobi, Kenya; the U.S. Naval Medical Research Center, Lima, Peru; the U.S. Naval Medical Research Unit, No. 2, Jakarta, Indonesia; and the U.S. Naval Medical Research Unit No. 3 in Cairo, Egypt. See the DoD-GEIS home page at http://www.geis.ha.osd.mil.

ical capabilities. The DoD facilities in Egypt and Indonesia have been designated as WHO Collaborating Centers for infectious disease.[11]

Electronic Surveillance System for Early Notification of Community-Based Epidemics (ESSENCE), a DoD-GEIS–administered, syndromic surveillance system that records outpatient diagnoses in eight syndrome categories from area military medical-treatment facilities.[12] Daily electronic dispatches of this information are compared to geographical and seasonal baselines.[13]

The Early Warning Outbreak Recognition System (EWORS), developed jointly by the U.S. Naval Medical Research Unit No. 2 in Jakarta, the Indonesian Ministry of Health, and the WHO, collects clinical data from five sentinel sites around Indonesia on a daily basis. The information is collected in Jakarta, where it is plotted geographically and analyzed.

Electronic Laboratory Reporting (ELR) is a means of reporting surveillance data and outbreak and other information from clinical laboratories to state health departments. In March 1997, the CDC, CSTE, and APHL met to determine recommended standards for ELR.[14] In 1998, Hawaii became the first state to establish a prototype for a statewide ELR system based on these recommendations. With assistance from the CDC, the Hawaii Department of Health (HDOH) developed a laboratory-based, electronic, communicable-disease reporting system, incorporating the state's three largest commercial

---

[11]Other WHO Collaborating Centers within DoD are USAMRIID, the Armed Forces Institute of Pathology's Department of Infectious and Parasitic Diseases Pathology, and the Division of Experimental Therapeutics at Walter Reed Army Institute of Research. GAO, "Global Health," July 20, 2000, p. 16.

[12]ESSENCE originally encompassed only the Washington, D.C., area (broadly defined) but it has now been expanded to cover the entire world. The population covered includes all those who go to military treatment facilities (active servicemembers, dependents, and retirees).

[13]Kelley, "Bioterrorism."

[14]Specifically, the CDC and CSTE recommended the adoption of Health Level 7 (HL7) as the standard format for electronic messages, Logical Observation Identifiers, Names and Codes as the standard for coding test names and the Systematized Nomenclature of Human and Veterinary Medicine as the standard for the test result codes. Greg Armstrong et al., "Electronic Reporting of Laboratory Information for Public Health, January 7–8, 1999, Summary of Proceedings," p. 1.

clinical laboratories. A study of this system published in the *Journal of the American Medical Association* (JAMA) compared the electronic system with conventional reporting by mail or fax and found that electronic reporting more than doubled the number of laboratory-based reports received by HDOH. Furthermore, the electronic reports were more complete and generally arrived several days before the conventional reports. The report concluded that if implemented nationwide, "ELR systems will likely have a positive impact on national morbidity figures and lead to a better understanding of communicable disease epidemiology. "[15]

The **Bio-Surveillance System**, although not a surveillance/data system per se, this $24 million, five-year DARPA project seeks to link disparate sources of health information to detect abnormal health events in the interest of protecting DoD personnel. The December 2000 project announcement referred to an earlier DARPA project that had mined grocery store, pharmacy, and absentee databases as well as healthcare records to detect an abnormal health event.[16]

INVESTIGATION ASSETS

The **Epidemic Intelligence Service (EIS)** carries out this direct support, known as Epidemiologic Assistance, or EPI-AIDs. EIS offers a two-year program in epidemiological training for physicians and public health specialists, emphasizing practical experience in field epidemiology.[17]

---

[15]Paul Effler et al., "Statewide System of Electronic Notifiable Disease Reporting from Clinical Laboratories: Comparing Automated Reporting with Conventional Methods," *JAMA*, Vol. 282, No. 19, November 17, 1999, pp. 1849–1850.

[16]Doug Brown, "Catching the Bug Before It Kills," *Interactive Week*, January 7, 2001, available at http://www.zdnet.com/intweek/stories/news/0,4164,2671596,00.html, accessed August 25, 2001. See also Murray Burke, "Bio-Surveillance System" slide presentation, available at http://www.darpa.mil/ito/research/rkfbio/biosurveillance_ito_web.pdf.

[17]The current annual EIS class size is about 70 students, a quarter of whom are placed in state or local health departments around the country. Stephen M. Ostroff, "The Epidemic Intelligence Service in the United States," *Eurosurveillance*, Vol. 6, No. 3, March 2001, pp. 34–36, available at http://www.ceses.org/eurosurveillance/V6n3/En53-222.htm, accessed August 13, 2001.

Laboratory Response Network (LRN) is a collaborative program between the CDC and the APHL that seeks to enhance laboratory capacity and diagnostic expertise for identifying and containing critical biological agents. Specifically, the LRN aims to develop screening and confirmation procedures for biological agents, expedite communication of test results, and facilitate transportation of specimens.

COMMUNICATION AND COORDINATION PROGRAMS

Information Network for Public Health Officials (INPHO) is a joint program between states and the CDC designed to help state health department officials to implement electronic information tools in support of public health objectives. Initiated in Georgia in 1993, INPHO has since awarded grants to 14 additional states. INPHO helps state public health departments to develop immunization registries, data warehousing, Internet access, and distance-based informatics training. INPHO also provided the groundwork for the information systems component of the Health Alert Network (see below).[18]

Health Alert Network (HAN) was launched by CDC's Public Health Practice Program Office in 1999. It aims to support local health agency efforts to track diseases, train public health professionals, and establish a standard, nationwide, information technology infrastructure to strengthen preparedness and response to bioterrorism and other public health emergencies.[19] When completed, HAN will enable electronic communication; delivery of health alerts from local health departments to the community; sharing of surveillance data, laboratory reports, and CDC diagnostic and treatment guidelines; and access by local health departments to CDC distance-learning programs. In 2000, the CDC funded cooperative agreements with 37 states, three counties, three cities, and two university research centers to build public health information technology capacity.[20] HAN also provides Secure Data Network, an Internet pipeline for encrypt-

---

[18]CDC, 2001 Program Review, p. 61.

[19]CDC, "Public Health's Infrastructure: A Status Report," p. 9.

[20]CDC, 2001 Program Review, p. 59.

ing and transferring files from health departments to the CDC. As of November 2000, 17 state surveillance systems were using Secure Data Network.[21]

Epidemic Information Exchange (Epi-X), which has been operational since November 2000, is a secure, Web-based communications network designed to expedite exchange of routine and emergency public health information between the CDC and state health departments.[22] Epi-X runs as an application on the HAN infrastructure, utilizes Secure Data Network, and is integrated with NEDSS.[23]

FOOD SAFETY INITIATIVES

The **Foodborne Disease Active Surveillance Network (FoodNet)** is a collaborative project involving the CDC, FDA, and USDA, is the food safety component of the EIP. FoodNet currently operates in nine states, monitoring 29 million people, or 11 percent of the U.S. population.[24] In addition to collecting information on all diarrheal illnesses in participating states, FoodNet has carried out surveys of laboratory and clinical practices with respect to foodborne illness diagnosis, as well as epidemiologic studies of *E. coli 0157:H7, Salmonella,* and *Campylobacter.*[25]

The **National Molecular Subtyping Network for Foodborne Disease Surveillance (PulseNet)** is a network of laboratories that perform DNA "fingerprinting" of bacteria believed to be foodborne using a method called pulsed-field gel electrophoresis. These molecular fingerprints are entered into an electronic database of other DNA fin-

---

[21]CDC, "Secure Data Network," available at http://www.cdc.gov/programs/research 22.htm, accessed August 15, 2001.

[22]CDC, "Epidemic Information Exchange (Epi-X)," available at http://www.cdc.gov/programs/research5.htm, accessed August 15, 2001.

[23]CSTE, "Support Development and Implementation of the Epidemiology Information Exchange," CSTE Position Statements 2000 EC-#4, available at http://www.cste.org/ps/2000/2000-ec-04.htm, accessed August 15, 2001.

[24]CDC, "Programs in Brief: Food Safety," available at http://www.cdc.gov/programs/environ6.htm, accessed August 15, 2001.

[25]CDC, "What Is FoodNet?" available at http://www.cdc.gov/foodnet/what_is.htm, accessed July 26, 2001.

gerprints at a state or local health department and compared with patterns in a database at CDC. Matching patterns from disparate sources during a given period of time indicate a possible multistate outbreak. In such cases, PulseNet sends e-mail alerts to all participating sites.[26] Forty-eight public health laboratories in 46 states currently participate in PulseNet.[27]

Hazard Analysis and Critical Control Point (HACCP) regulations, issued in 1996 by FSIS, require hazard analysis to identify critical points in the food production process and the application of preventive and corrective measures aimed at eliminating hazards at those points.[28] HACCP represents a shift in FSIS's regulatory approach to include the production process as well as the finished product.[29] Implementation of the HACCP system was completed in 2000.

The **National Antimicrobial Monitoring System (NARMS) for Enteric Bacteria** is a surveillance system for tracking changes in antimicrobial susceptibility in humans and food animals. It was initiated in 1996 by HHS and USDA and expanded under the auspices of the FoodNet system.[30] Human-origin isolates of *Salmonella, Shigella,* and *E. coli 0157:H7* are sent by 17 state and local health departments to the CDC. Eight participating departments also submit *Campylobacter* isolates on a weekly basis.[31] Animal-origin isolates are sent from FSIS, the USDA/APHIS National Animal Health Monitoring System, and National Veterinary Services laboratories and sentinel sites to the USDA's Agricultural Research Service laboratory in Athens,

---

[26]CDC, "PulseNet: The National Molecular Subtyping Network for Foodborne Disease Surveillance," available at http://www.cdc.gov/ncidod/dbmd/pulsenet/pulsenet.htm, accessed July 11, 2001.

[27]CDC, "Programs in Brief: Food Safety."

[28]FDA, "HAACP."

[29]USDA/FSIS, "Protecting the Public From Foodborne Illness."

[30]Participating agencies include the following: FDA, Center for Veterinary Medicine; CDC; FSIS, Agricultural Research Service; and APHIS.

[31]Participating health departments are those in California, Colorado, Connecticut, Florida, Georgia, Kansas, Los Angeles County, Maryland, Minnesota, Massachusetts, New Jersey, New York City, New York, Oregon, Tennessee, Washington, and West Virginia. Connecticut, Georgia, Maryland, Minnesota, New York, Oregon, and Tennessee also submit *Campylobacter* isolates. Center for Veterinary Medicine, FDA, "National Antimicrobial Resistance Monitoring System-Enteric Bacteria," available at http://www.fda.gov/cvm/index/narms/narmsbro.htm, accessed August 15, 2001.

Georgia. Human- and animal-origin isolates are tested for susceptibility to 17 antimicrobial agents. *Campylobacter* isolates are tested
for susceptibility to eight antimicrobial agents.

RESPONSE

The **Chemical and Biological Rapid Response Team (CB-RRT)** is a
joint unit developed from DoD chemical and biological assets,
including the U.S. Army Technical Escort Unit, the Army 52nd Ord-
nance Group, USAMRIID, U.S. Army Medical Research Institute for
Chemical Defense, Edgewood CB Forensic Analytical Center, the
Navy Medical Research Institute, Navy Environmental and Preventive Medicine Unit, and Navy Research Laboratory. The Technical
Escort Unit is the lead element of the CB-RRT and can deploy a 12-
person CB-RRT nationwide within four hours of notification.

The **Chemical and Biological Incident Response Force (CBIRF)**,
activated in 1996, is a Marine Corps unit based at the Naval Surface
Warfare Center (NSWC) with chemical and biological terrorism
consequence-management capabilities.[32] Although CBIRF's primary
mission is to respond to attacks on U.S. Navy and State Department
facilities worldwide, the unit may be deployed for a domestic incident in support of local authorities and the OEP.[33] CBIRF is composed of approximately 375 personnel organized into command and
control, reconnaissance, decontamination, medical, security, and
service support elements. This unit has capabilities to detect and
identify chemical and biological agents, and evacuate, decontami-
nate, triage, and treat patients.[34]

The **National Disaster Medical System (NDMS)** is an asset-sharing
partnership among HHS, DoD, FEMA, the Department of Veterans
Affairs, state and local governments, private businesses, and civilian

---

[32]Smithson and Levy, *Ataxia*, p. 138.

[33]Jonathan B. Tucker, "National Health and Medical Services Response to Incidents of
Chemical and Biological Terrorism," *JAMA*, Vol. 278, No. 5, 1997, pp. 362–368, available at http://www.lsic.ucla.edu/classes/mimg/spring01/micro12/Website/JAMA
articles/response.html, accessed July 5, 2001.

[34]Koblentz, p. 31.

volunteers.[35] The NDMS is designed to provide integrated national medical assistance during major peacetime disasters within 12 hours.[36] More than 7,000 NDMS volunteer health professionals are organized into 80 Disaster Medical Assistance Teams.[37] NDMS also includes Disaster Mortuary Operations Response Teams and Veterinary Medical Assistance Teams. The NDMS capability includes the provision of in-hospital care for up to 100,000 victims.[38]

The **National Immunization Program (NIP)** of the CDC provides leadership for the planning, coordination, and institution of immunization activities nationwide. It is subdivided into four main divisions—Data Management, Epidemiology and Surveillance, Immunization Services, and Global Immunization—and currently oversees seven vaccine-related areas.[39] The NIP was preceded by the National Vaccine Program Office (NVPO), which was an attempt during the early part of the Clinton administration to coordinate HHS immunization programs.[40]

---

[35]HHS, Office of Emergency Preparedness home page, available at http://www. oep.dhhs.gov/, accessed July 6, 2001.

[36]HHS, Office of Emergency Preparedness, "NDMS: Catastrophic Care for the Nation," available at http://ndms.dhhs.gov/NDMS/ndms.html, accessed July 2, 2001. NDMS has three components: direct medical care, patient evacuation, and non-federal hospital care. HHS, "Medical Response in Emergencies: HHS Role," fact sheet, January 25, 2001, available at http://www.os.dhhs.gov/news/press/2001pres/01fs emergencyresponse.html, accessed July 6, 2001.

[37]HHS, "Medical Response in Emergencies."

[38]Tommy G. Thompson, Secretary, HHS, testimony before the Subcommittee on Commerce, Justice, State, and Judiciary, Committee on Appropriations, U.S. Senate, May 9, 2001, available at http://www.os.dhhs.gov/progorg/asl/testify/t010509.html, accessed September 3, 2001.

[39]These include child vaccines, vaccine safety, tracking vaccine-preventable diseases, measles immunization, immunization grant programs, development of immunization registries, and adult/adolescent immunization. For further details, see http://www. cdc.gov/nip/.

[40]CDC, "About NVPO," available at http://www.cdc.gov/od/nvpo/who.htm.

BIBLIOGRAPHY

Abshire, David, "US Foreign Policy in the Post Cold War Era: The Need for an Agile Strategy," *Washington Quarterly,* Vol. 19, No. 2, 1996, pp. 42–44.

Advisory Panel to Assess Domestic Response Capabilities for Terrorism Involving Weapons of Mass Destruction, *First Annual Report to the President and the Congress—I: Assessing the Threat,* Santa Monica, Calif.: RAND, December 15, 1999.

_____, *Second Annual Report to the President and the Congress—II: Toward a National Strategy for Combating Terrorism,* Santa Monica, Calif.: RAND, December 15, 2000.

"AIDS Wipes Out [South Africa's] Teachers," *Sunday Times* (South Africa), December 14, 2001; and "AIDS Wipes Out [South Africa's] Teachers," *Sunday Times* (South Africa) (Internet version), available at http://www.suntimes.co.za/2001/11/94/news/news02. osp, accessed January 10, 2001.

Alibek, Ken, *Biohazard,* New York: Random House, 1999.

Altman, Lawrence K., "A Nation Challenged: NBC; Doctor in City Reported Anthrax Case Before Florida," *New York Times,* October, 18, 2001, p. B7.

American Society for Microbiology, "List of Currently Known BSL-4 Facilities Worldwide," available at http://www.asmusa.org/memonly/asmnews/nov99/figs/t1f1.htm, accessed July 12, 2001.

_____, Clinical Microbiology Issues Update, "ASM Submits Testimony to Congress," April 2001, available at http://www. asmusa.org/pasrc/clinicalmicro-april2001.htm, accessed June 22, 2002.

Animal and Plant Health Inspection Service (APHIS), "International Services," available at http://www.aphis.usda.gov/is/, accessed August 17, 2001.

"Antibiotic Resistant Germ Kills Woman, Hong Kong Officials Say," CNN Interactive World Wide News, February 22, 1999.

Armelagos, George, "The Viral Superhighway," *The Sciences*, Vol. 38, No. 1, 1998.

Armstrong, Greg, Scott Danos, Ron Fichtner, Joy Herndon, Dan Jernigan, Denise Koo, Carol Pertowski, Robert Pinner, Steve Steindel, Suzanne Sutlift, Jac Davies, Ralph Timperi, and Susan Toal, "Electronic Reporting of Laboratory Information for Public Health, January 7–8, 1999, Summary of Proceedings," p. 1.

Arndt, Channing, and Jeffrey Lewis, "The Macro Implications of HIV/AIDS in South Africa: A Preliminary Assessment," The World Bank, August 2000, available at http://www.worldbank.org/afr/wps/wp9.pdf.

Asian Development Bank (ADB), "Rise of the Megacity," April 24, 1997.

Associated Press, "S. Africa Sued for Failing to Distribute AIDS Drug," *Washington Post*, August 22, 2001, p. A14.

Atlas, Ronald, "Combating the Threat of Biowarfare and Bioterrorism: Defending Against Biological Weapons Is Critical to Global Security," *Bioscience*, Vol. 49, No. 5, 1999.

Axeworthy, Lloyd, "Human Security: Safety for People in a Changing World," Department of Foreign Affairs and International Trade, Ottawa, April 1999.

Becker, Elizabeth, and Robin Toner, "A Nation Challenged: The Victims, Postal Workers' Illness Set Off No Alarms," *New York Times*, October 24, 2001, p. B1.

Benatar, Solomon, "South Africa's Transition in a Globalizing World: HIV/AIDS as a Window and Mirror," *International Affairs,* Vol. 77, No. 2, 2001.

Berry, Marsha, and Lawrence Gostin, "Model Emergency Health Powers Act in Response to Bioterrorism Written for the CDC and Governors: Act to Help Ensure Rapid and Orderly Response to Public Health Threats," Georgetown University Law Center, October 30, 2001, available at http://www.law.georgetown.edu/topics/releases/october.30.2001.html.

Bill and Melinda Gates Foundation, "The Bill and Melinda Gates Foundation Announces New HIV/AIDS Grants at World AIDS Conference," press release, July 12, 2000, available at http://www.gatesfoundation.org/pressroom/release.asp?Prindex=245.

_____, "Pledges US$100 Million Toward $550 Million AIDS Vaccine Goal," press release, January 27, 2001, available at http://www.gatesfoundation.org/pressroom/release.asp?Prindex=344.

"Bin Laden Goes After Big Guns," NBC Interactive News, June 15, 2000, available at http://www.msnbc.com/news/421013.

Blatz, W. E., *Human Security: Some Reflections,* Toronto: University of Toronto Press, 1966.

Blommer Anne, et al., "Women's Issues in South Africa," available at http://www.evergreen.edu/users6/menste01/gender.html.

Brown, Bruce, Scott Dowell, Alexandra Levitt, and James M. Hughes, "Setting Priorities for Global Infectious Disease Control," *U.S. Medicine,* April 2001, available at http://www.usmedicine.com/column.cfm?columnID=44&issueID=25, accessed July 6, 2001.

Brown, Doug, "Catching the Bug Before It Kills," *Interactive Week,* January 7, 2001, available at http://www.zdnet.com/intweek/stories/news/0,4164,2671596,00.html, accessed August 25, 2001.

Brown, Seyom, "World Interests and the Changing Dimensions of World Security," in Michael Klare and Daniel Thomas, eds., *World Security: Challenges for a New Century,* New York: St. Martin's Press, 1994, pp. 10–26.

Buerhaus, P., D. Staiger, and D. Auerbach, "Implications of an Aging Registered Nurse Workforce," *JAMA*, Vol. 283, No. 22, June 14, 2000, pp. 2948–2954.

Burke, Murray, "Bio-Surveillance System" slide presentation, available at http://www.darpa.mil/ito/research/rkfbio/biosurveil lance_ito_web.pdf .

Calling the Shots, Committee on Immunization Finance Policies and Practices, Division of Health Care Services and Division of Health Promotion and Disease Prevention, Institute of Medicine, National Academy Press, Washington, D.C., 2000.

Carus, Seth, *Bioterrorism and Biocrimes: The Illicit Use of Biological Agents in the 20th Century,* Washington, D.C.: Center for Counterproliferation Research, National Defense University, 1999.

Center for Strategic and International Studies (CSIS), *Contagion and Conflict: Health as a Global Security Challenge,* Washington, D.C.: 2000.

Center for Veterinary Medicine, FDA, "National Antimicrobial Resistance Monitoring System-Enteric Bacteria," available at http://www.fda.gov/cvm/index/narms/narmsbro.htm, accessed August 15, 2001.

Centers for Disease Control and Prevention (CDC), "Addressing Emerging Infectious Disease Threats: A Prevention Strategy for the United States," Atlanta: CDC, 1994.

_____, "Public Health's Infrastructure: A Status Report," p. 9.

_____, "About NVPO," available at http://www.cdc.gov/od/nvpo/who.htm.

_____, "Preventing Emerging Infectious Diseases: A Strategy for the 21st Century," Atlanta: CDC, October 1998.

_____, "Border Infectious Disease Surveillance Project Moves Forward," *NCID Focus*, Vol. 1, No. 2, March–April 2000, p. 4.

_____, "Towards a National Laboratory System," November 2000, p. 3, available at http://www.phppo.cdc.gov/mlp/pdf/nls/nls.1101.pdf, accessed August 3, 2001.

_____, 2001 Program Review, "National Laboratory Network," press kit, available at www.cdc.gov/od/oc/media/presskit/training.htm.

_____, "Economic Costs for Patient Care from Infectious Diseases, United States," available at http://www.cdc.gov/ncidod/emerg plan/box02.htm.

_____, "Surveillance Resources: Surveillance Systems," available at http://www.cdc.ncidod/osr/survsyss.htm, accessed July 3, 2001.

_____, "Surveillance Systems Home Pages and Contacts," available at http://www.cdc.gov/ncidod/osr/survsyss.htm#EMERGE, accessed July 3, 2001.

_____, "NPS Synopsis," available at http://www.cdc.gov/nceh/nps/synopses.htm, accessed July 6, 2001.

_____, "Supporting Public Health Surveillance Through the National Electronic Disease Surveillance System (NEDSS)," available at http://www.cdc.gov/od/hissb/docs/NEDSS%20Intro.pdf, accessed July 6, 2001.

_____, "Epidemiology and Laboratory Capacity (ELC) for Infectious Diseases Cooperative Agreement," available at http://www.cdc.gov/ncidod/osr/ELC.htm, accessed July 11, 2001.

_____, "PulseNet: The National Molecular Subtyping Network for Foodborne Disease Surveillance," available at http://www.cdc.gov/ncidod/dbmd/pulsenet/pulsenet.htm, accessed July 11, 2001.

_____, "About Epi-Info," available at http://www.cdc.gov/epiinfo/aboutepi.htm, accessed July 12, 2001.

_____, "What Is FoodNet?" available at http://www.cdc.gov/foodnet/what_is.htm, accessed July 26, 2001.

_____, "National Center for Infectious Disease (HCR)," available at http://www.cdc.gov/maso/ncidfs.htm, accessed August 3, 2001.

_____, "Enhanced Surveillance Project (ESP)," available at http://www.bt.cdc.gov/EpiSurv/ESP.asp, accessed August 8, 2001.

_____, "Requests for Epidemiologic Assistance (EPI-AIDs)," available at http://www.cdc.gov/programs/partners9.htm, accessed August 15, 2001.

_____, "About NIP," available at www.cdc.gov/nip/about/, accessed August 15, 2001.

_____, "Disease Information: Typhoid Fever," available at http://www.cdc.gov/ncidod/dbmd/diseaseinfo/typhoidfever_g.htm.

_____, "Epidemic Information Exchange (Epi-X)," available at http://www.cdc.gov/programs/research5.htm, accessed August 15, 2001.

_____, "Guide to Community Preventive Services," available at http://www.cdc.gov/programs/partners4.htm, accessed August 15, 2001.

_____, "International Training Programs for Applied Epidemiology and Global Health Leadership," available at http://www.cdc.gov/programs/global5.htm, accessed August 15, 2001.

_____, "Prevention Guidelines," available at http://wonder.cdc.gov/wonder/prevguid/library/library.asp, accessed August 15, 2001.

_____, "Programs in Brief: Food Safety," available at http://www.cdc.gov/programs/environ6.htm, accessed August 15, 2001.

_____, "Secure Data Network," available at http://www.cdc.gov/programs/research22.htm, accessed August 15, 2001.

_____, "What Is NARMS?" available at http://www.cdc.gov/ncidod/dbmd/narms/what_is.htm, accessed August 16, 2001.

_____, "National Immunization Program: Vaccines for Children," available at http://www.cdc.gov/nip/vfc/Parent/ParentHome Page.htm, accessed August 27, 2001.

_____, "Antibiotic Resistance," available at Http://www.cdc.gov/antibioticresistance/, accessed June 21, 2002.

CDC and ATSDR, "Working with Partners to Improve Global Health: A Strategy for CDC and ATSDR," September 2000, p. 4, available at www.cdc.gov/ogh/pub/execsummary.pdf.

CDC–National Center for HIV, STD, and TB Prevention–Division of HIV/AIDS Prevention, "HIV/AIDS Surveillance Supplemental Reports," available at http://www.cdc.gov/hiv/stats/hasrsupp51. htm.

Central Intelligence Agency, *Report 2000: The Global Infectious Disease Threat and Its Implications for the United States,* available at http://www.cia.gov/cia/publications/nie/report/nie99-17d.html, pp. 6, 33.

Chalk, Peter, "Low Intensity Conflict in Southeast Asia," *Conflict Studies,* Vol. 305, No. 306, 1998, p. 12.

_____, *Non-Military Security and Global Order: The Impact of Violence, Chaos and Disorder on International Security,* London: Macmillan, 2000.

"Changing Climate," *The Australian,* July 15, 1996.

Chemical and Biological Arms Control Institute and the CSIS International Security Program, *Contagion and Conflict: Health as a Global Security Challenge,* Washington, D.C.: CSIS, January 2000, p. 3.

Chiles, Nick, "Major Screening for TB Shows Contrast in Conditions Since Days of Ellis Island," *New York Times* online, January 11, 2000, available at http://www.nytimes.com/learning/teachers/featured_articles/20000111tuesday.html, accessed December 15, 2001.

"Chinese City Portrays Good and Bad of Rapid Growth," *Bangkok Post,* December 10, 1997.

Chivian, E., "Microorganisms, Disease and Security, Technology, Social Change, Demography," *Technology Review,* November/December 1994.

Chow, Jack, "Health and International Security," *Washington Quarterly,* Vol. 19, No. 2, 1996.

Cifuentes, L., V. H. Borja-Aburto, N. Gouveia, G. Thurston, and D. L. Davis, "Hidden Health Benefits of Greenhouse Gas Mitigation," *Science,* August 17, 2001, Vol. 293, pp. 1257–1259.

"Cleaning Up in Asia," *The Australian,* May 19, 1997.

CNN, "FDA Approves First in a Long-Awaited New Class of Antibiotics," April 18, 2000, available at www.cnn.co/2000/HEALTH/04/18/new.antibiotic, accessed December 7, 2000.

_____, "Antibiotic Resistance a Growing Threat," June 12, 2000, available at http://www.cnn.com/2000/health/06/12/antibiotic.resistance, accessed June 21, 2002.

Cohen, Mitchell, "Changing Patterns of Infectious Disease," *Nature,* Vol. 406, 2000, pp. 762–767.

Colvin, Mark, and Eleanor Gouws, "Thukela Water Project Feasibility Study: An Assessment of HIV/AIDS—Its Context and Implications for the TWP," paper provided to the author, August 2001.

Colvin, Mark, and Brian Sharp, "Communicable Diseases and Poverty in Southern Africa," paper presented at a South Afrrican Regional Policy Network Conference at Human Sciences Research Council, Pretoria, April 26, 2001, pp. 4–5.

Committee on HIV Prevention Strategies in the United States, *No Time to Lose: Getting More From HIV Prevention,* Washington, D.C.: The Institute of Medicine, 2001.

Council of State and Territorial Epidemiologists (CSTE), "Support Development and Implementation of the Epidemiology Information Exchange," CSTE Position Statements 2000 EC-#4, available at http://www.cste.org/ps/2000/2000-ec-04.htm, accessed August 15, 2001.

"Cruelest Curse, The," *The Economist,* February 24, 2001.

Crabb, Charlene, "Hard-Won Advances Spark Excitement About Hepatitis C," *Science,* Vol. 294, 2001, pp. 506–507.

Dalby, Simon, "Security, Intelligence, the National Interest and the Global Environment," *Intelligence and National Security,* Vol. 10, No. 4, 1995, p. 186.

Davis, Jonathan R., and Joshua Lederberg, eds., *Public Health Systems and Emerging Infections: Assessing the Capabilities of the*

Public and Private Sectors—Workshop Summary, Washington, D.C.: National Academy Press, 2001, p. 6.

Day, Karen, "Malaria: A Global Threat," in Richard Krause, ed., *Emerging Infections,* New York: Academic Press, 1998, p. 485.

"Deadly Ebola Bug Strikes Uganda," *The New Straits Times,* October 18, 2000.

Department of Finance (South Africa), *Budget Review 2000,* Pretoria: Department of Finance, 2000, p. 29.

Department of Health (South Africa), National HIV and Syphilis Sero-Prevalence Survey of Women Attending Public Antenatal Clinics in South Africa, 2000, available at http://www.doh.gov.za/docs/reports/2000/hivreport.html.

Dewar, Helen, "Senate Bioterrorism Bill Doubles Bush's Request," *Washington Post,* November 16, 2001, p. A15.

Dircks, Ruth, ed., *Disease and Society: A Resource Book,* Canberra: Australian Academy of Science, 1989.

"Disease Threatens Survivors," *The Australian,* November 9, 1998.

Division of Laboratory Systems, available at http://www.phppo.cdc.gov/mlp/nls.asp, accessed August 13, 2001.

Dupont, Alan, "Regional Security Concerns into the 21st Century," in John Ciccarelli, ed., *Transnational Crime: A New Security Threat?* Canberra: Australian Defence Studies Centre, pp. 72–73.

Earnest, Mark, and John Sbarbaro, "A Plague Returns," *The Sciences,* Vol. 33, No. 5, September/October 1993, pp. 17–18.

Ebhert, Dave, "Model State Bioterror Law Stirs Controversy," Vaccine Information Center, January 3, 2002, available at http://www.vaclib.org/legal/invol.htm.

Effler, Paul, Myrna Chinj-Lee, April Bogard, Man-Cheng Leong, Trudi Nekomoto, and Daniel Jernigan, "Statewide System of Electronic Notifiable Disease Reporting from Clinical Laboratories: Comparing Automated Reporting with Conventional Methods," *JAMA,* Vol. 282, No. 19, November 17, 1999, pp. 1849–1850.

Epstein, P., "Emerging Diseases and Ecosystem Instability: New Threats to Public Health," *American Journal of Public Health*, Vol. 85, 1995.

Epstein, Paul, "Climate and Health," *Science*, Vol. 285, 1999, pp. 347–348.

"Euro-Atlantic Relationship: Ready for the Global Era?" Wilton Park Conference, Wilton Park, UK, May 21–25, 2001.

Falkenrath, Richard, "Confronting Nuclear, Biological and Chemical Terrorism," *Survival*, Vol. 40, No. 3, 1998, pp. 45–46.

_____, Robert Newman, and Brad Thayer, *America's Achilles' Heel: Nuclear, Biological and Chemical Terrorism and Covert Attack*, Cambridge, Mass.: MIT Press, 1998.

"Fatal Human Plague—Arizona and Colorado, 1996," *MMWR*, Vol. 46, No. 27, July 11, 1997, pp. 617–620.

Fauci, A., and T. Quinn, "The AIDS Epidemic: Considerations for the 21st Century," *New England Journal of Medicine*, Vol. 341, No. 14, 1999.

Fauci, Anthony S., Director, NIAID, statement before the Subcommittee on Labor, Health and Human Services, and Education, U.S. House of Representatives, May 16, 2001, available at http://www.niaid.nih.gov/director/congress/2001/051601.htm, accessed August 28, 2001.

Federal Bureau of Investigation, *Crime in the United States, 1996*, Washington, D.C.: Department of Justice, 1996.

Federal Emergency Management Agency, "FPR . . . at a Glance," available at http://www.fema.gov/r-n-r/frp/frpglnc.htm, accessed July 10, 2001.

"Fever Kills 200 in Saudi Arabia and Yemen," Reuters, September 24, 2000.

FitzSimons, D. W., and A. W. Whiteside, "Conflict, War and Public Health," *Conflict Studies*, Vol. 276, 1994.

Food and Drug Administration (FDA), "Food and Drug Administration Recall Policies," available at http://vm.cfsan.fda.gov/~lrd/recall2.html.

_____, "HACCP: A State-of-the-Art Approach to Food Safety," August 1999, available at http://vm.cfsan.fda.gov/~lrd/bghaccp.html, accessed July 26, 2001.

FDA, USDA, U.S. Environmental Protection Agency, and CDC, "Food Safety from Farm to Table: A National Food Safety Initiative," report to the President, May 1997, available at http://www.cdc.gov/ncidod/foodsafe/report.htm, accessed August 3, 2001.

Food Safety Inspection Service (FSIS), "Food Recalls," available at http://www.fsis.usda.gov/OA/pubs/recallfocus.htm.

Foreman, C. H., Jr., *Plagues, Products, and Politics: Emergent Public Health Hazards and National Policymaking*, Washington, D.C.: Brookings Institution Press, 1994.

Foster, S., and S. Lucas, *Socioeconomic Aspects of HIV and AIDS in Developing Countries: A Review and Annotated Bibliography*, Public Health Policy Departmental Publication No. 3, London: London School of Hygiene and Tropical Medicine, 1991.

Garrett, L., *Betrayal of Trust: The Collapse of Global Public Health*, New York: Hyperion Press, 2000.

Garrett, Laurie, *The Coming Plague: Newly Emerging Diseases in a World out of Balance*, New York: Penguin Books, 1994.

_____, "The Return of Infectious Disease," *Foreign Affairs*, Vol. 75, No. 1, January/February 1996.

_____, "Gates Urges More Funds for HIV Prevention," *Washington Post*, April 8, 2001, p. A5.

Gellman, Barton, "Unequal Calculus of Life and Death, An," *Washington Post*, December 27, 2000, p. A1.

General Accounting Office (GAO), "Emerging Infectious Diseases: Consensus on Needed Laboratory Capacity Could Strengthen Surveillance," GAO/HEHS-99-26, February 1999, p. 7.

_____, "Emerging Infectious Diseases: National Surveillance System Could Be Strengthened," GAO/T-HEHS-99-62, February 25, 1999, p. 4.

_____, "Global Health: Framework for Infectious Disease Surveillance," GAO/NSIAD-00-205R, July 20, 2000.

_____, "West Nile Virus Outbreak: Lessons for Public Health Preparedness," GAO/HEHS-00-180, September 2000.

George Washington University, "Preparing for a Bioterrorist Incident: Linking the Public Health and Medical Communities," National Health Policy Forum, October 4–5, 1999, site visit to Baltimore and Fort Detrick, Md.

Giddens, Anthony, *The Consequences of Modernity: Self and Society in the Late Modern Age,* Stanford, Calif.: Stanford University Press, 1990.

"Global Infectious Disease Threat and Its Implications for the United States, The," *Foreign Affairs,* Vol. 75, No. 1, January/February 1998, p. 23.

Gostin, Lawrence, Z. Lazzarini, V. S. Neslund, and M. T. Osterholm, "Water Quality Laws and Watreborne Diseases: Cryptosporidium and Other Emerging Pathogens," *American Journal of Public Health,* Vol. 90, 2000, pp. 847–853.

Graham, J., and B. Bowling, *Young People and Crime,* Home Office Research Study No. 145, London: Her Majesty's Stationery Office, 1995.

Gregg, M., ed., *The Public Health Consequences of Disasters,* Atlanta: CDC, 1989.

Harvell, C. D., C. E. Mitchell, J. R. Ward, S. Alitzer, P. Dobson, R. S. Ostfeld, and M. D. Samuel, "Climate Warming and Disease Risks for Terrestrial and Marine Biota," *Science,* June 21, 2002, pp. 2158–2162.

"Health of Nations, The," *The Economist,* December 22, 2001.

Health Systems Trust (South Africa), "South African Health Review 2000," available at http://www.hsat.org/za/sahr/2000.

Heinecken, Lindy, "HIV/AIDS, the Military and the Impact on National and International Security," paper presented at the millennium colloquium of the South African Political Studies Association, Bloemfontein, South Africa, September 20–22, 2000.

_____, "Strategic Implications of HIV/AIDS in South Africa," *Journal of Conflict and Development*, Vol. 1, No. 1, 2001.

Heinrich, Janet, "Health Workforce: Ensuring Adequate Supply and Distribution Remains Challenging," Washington, D.C.: GAO, August 1, 2001.

Henderson, D., T. V. Inglesby, J. G. Bartlett, M. S. Ascher, E. Eitzen, P. B. Jahrling, J. Hauer, M. Layton, J. McDade, M. T. Osterholm, T. O'Toole, G. Parker, T. Perl, P. K. Russell, and K. Tonat, for the Working Group on Civilian Biodefense, "Smallpox as a Biological Weapon: Medical and Public Health Management," *JAMA*, Vol. 281, No. 22, 1999.

"HIV and AIDS—United States, 1981–2000," *MMWR*, Vol. 50, No. 21, June 1, 2001, pp. 430–434.

"HIV Incidence Among Young Men Who Have Sex with Men—Seven US Cities, 1994–2000," *MMWR*, Vol. 50, No. 21, 2001, pp. 440–444.

Hjelle, Brian, "Hantaviruses, with Emphasis on Four Corners Hantavirus," 1996, available at http://www.bocklabs.wisc.edu/ed/hanta.html, accessed November 16, 2001.

Hoffman, Bruce, "Twenty-First Century Terrorism," foreword in James M. Smith and William C. Thomas, eds., *The Terrorism Threat and the U.S. Government Response: Operational and Organizational Factors*, Colorado Springs, Colo.: U.S. Air Force Institute for National Security Studies, 2001.

Holden-Rhodes, Jim, and Peter Lupsha, "Gray Area Phenomena: New Threats and Policy Dilemmas," *Criminal Justice International*, Vol. 9, No. 1, 1993, pp. 11–17.

_____, "Horsemen of the Apocalypse: Gray Area Phenomena and the New World Disorder," *Low Intensity Conflict and Law Enforcement*, Vol. 2, No. 2, 1993, pp. 212–226.

Holmberg, S. D., "The Estimated Prevalence and Incidence of HIV in 96 Large US Metropolitan Areas," *American Journal of Public Health*, Vol. 86, No. 5, 1996, pp. 642–654.

Home Office Research and Statistics Department, "Information on the Criminal Justice System in England and Wales," London: Her Majesty's Stationery Office, 1995.

Houghton, J. T., Y. Ding, D. J. Griggs, M. Nouger, P. J. van der Linden, and D. Xiaosou, eds., *IPCC Third Assessment Report: Climate Change 2001—The Scientific Basis*, available at http://www.ipcc.ch/pub/reports.htm.

Hughes, James M., M.D., Director, National Center for Infectious Diseases, CDC, HHS, testimony before the Subcommittee on National Security, Veterans Affairs, and International Relations, Committee on Government Reform, U.S. House of Representatives, May 1, 2001, available at http://www.hhs.gov.asl/testify/t010501a.html, accessed July 9, 2001.

Infectious Disease Society of America, "Emerging Infections Network," available at http://www.idsociety.org/EIN/TOC.htm, accessed July 11, 2001.

_____ "Emerging Infections Network: Background and Organization," available at www.idsociety.org/EIN/AboutEIN.htm, accessed July 27, 2001.

ING Barings, *Economic Impact of AIDS in South Africa: A Dark Cloud on the Horizon*, London: ING Barings, April 2000.

Institute of Medicine (IOM), Committee for the Study of the Future of Public Health, Division of Health Care Services, *The Future of Public Health*, Washington, D.C.: National Academy Press, 1988.

_____, "Public Health Systems and Emerging Infections: Assessing the Capabilities of the Public and Private Sectors, Workshop Summary," Washington, D.C.: National Academy Press, 2000.

International Monetary Fund, *The World Economic Outlook*, Washington, D.C., 1991.

International Society of Travel Medicine, "GeoSentinel: Objectives," available at http://www.istm.org/geosweb/objectiv.html, accessed August 7, 2001.

Jackson, Ronald J., Alistair J. Ramsay, Carolina D. Christensen, Sandra Beaton, Diana F. Hall, and Ian A. Ramshaw, "Expression of Mouse Interleukin-4 by a Recombinant Ectromelia Virus Suppresses Cytolytic Lymphocyte Responses and Overcomes Genetic Resistance to Mousepox," *Journal of Virology,* Vol. 75, No. 3, February 2001, pp. 1205–1210.

"Japan Declares E. coli Epidemic an Outbreak: Citizens Accuse Government of Slow Response," CNN Interactive World Wide News, August 1, 1996.

"Keeping China's Blood Supply Free of HIV/AIDS," U.S. Embassy, April 1997, available at http://www.usembassy-china.org.cn/english/sandt/webaids5.htm, accessed on March 13, 2002.

Kelley, Col. Patrick, "Bioterrorism: Alert and Response," available at http://cer.hs.washington.edu/em_inf/bio/bio.html, accessed August 31, 2001.

Kimball, Ann Marie, "Overview and Surveillance of Emerging Infections," available at http://cer.hs.washington.edu/em_inf/emerging/cmerg.html, accessed September 3, 2001.

Kinghorn, A., and M. Steinberg, "HIV/AIDS in South Africa: The Impact and the Priorities," Department of Health (South Africa) document (undated), p. 14, cited in Martin Schönteich, "AIDS and Age: SA's Crime Time Bomb?" *AIDS Analysis Africa,* Vol. 10, No. 2, 1999. p. 1.

Knobler, S.L., A. A. F. Mahmoud, and L. A. Pray, eds., "Vaccines Research, Development, Production and Procurement Issues," in *Biological Threats and Terrorism: Assessing the Science and Response Capabilities,* Forum on Emerging Infections, Board on Global Health, 2002, pp. 85–121;

Koblentz, Gregory D., "Overview of Federal Programs to Enhance State and Local Preparedness for Terrorism with Weapons of Mass Destruction," Belfer Center for Science and International Affairs Discussion Paper 2001-5, Executive Session on Domestic Preparedness Discussion Paper ESDP-2001-3, Cambridge, Mass.: John F. Kennedy School of Government, Harvard University, April 2001.

Kolata, G., "Clues to Deadly Virus Changes Seen," *San Jose Mercury News*, September 7, 2001, available at www.mercurycenter.com/ cgi-bin/edtoolssss/printpage/printpage_ba.cgi, accessed September 7, 2001.

Kondrachine, A., "Mission Report on Malaria Epidemics in Rajasthan," unpublished World Health Organization (WHO) Report, 1996.

_____, "Malaria in Peru," unpublished WHO report, 1997.

_____, and P. Trigg, "Global Overview of Malaria," *Indian Journal of Medical Research*, Vol. 106, 1997, pp. 39–53.

Krause, Keith, and Michael Williams, "From Strategy to Security: Foundations of Critical Security Studies," in Keith Krause and Michael Williams, eds., *Critical Security Studies*, Minneapolis: University of Minnesota Press, 1997, p. 43.

Last, John, *Public Health and Human Ecology*, Stamford, Conn.: Appleton and Lange, 1998.

Latter, Richard, "Terrorism in the 1990s," *Wilton Park Papers*, Vol. 44, 1991, p. 2.

Lechat, M., "The Epidemiology of Health Effects of Disasters," *Epidemiological Review*, Vol. 12, 1990.

Lederberg, Joshua, ed., *Biological Weapons: Limiting the Threat*, Cambridge, Mass.: MIT Press, 1999.

_____, comments made during the International Conference on Emerging Infectious Diseases (ICEID), Atlanta, Ga., July 16–19, 2000.

Lepers J., D. Fontenville, M. D. Rason, C. Chougnet, P. Astagneau, P. Coulanges, and P. Deloron "Transmission and Epidemiology of Newly Transmitted Falciparum Malaria in the Central Highland Plateau of Madagascar," *Annals of Tropical Medicine*, Vol. 85, 1991, pp. 297–304.

Levy, S. B., *The Antibiotic Paradox: How the Misuse of Antibiotics Destroys Their Curative Powers*, 2nd edition, Cambridge, Mass.: Perseus Publishing, 2002.

Levy, Stuart B., "The Challenge of Antibiotic Resistance," *Scientific American*, Vol. 278, No. 3, March 1998, pp. 46–53.

_____, American Society for Microbiology, "Antibiotic Resistance: Microbes on the Defense," in *Congressional Briefing: Infectious Diseases as We Enter the New Century: What Can We Do?* June 21, 1999, p. 5.

Lillibridge, Scott, comments made during the Biological and Chemical Preparedness: The New Challenge for Public Health meeting, Decatur, Ill., July 19–20, 2000.

Lillie-Blanton, M., and J. Hudman, "Untangling the Web: Race/Ethnicity, Immigration, and the Nation's Health," *American Journal of Public Health*, Vol. 91, No. 11, November 2001, p. 1736.

"Limits of $100 Million, The," *Washington Post*, December 29, 2000, p. A1.

Linden, Eugene, "The Exploding Cities of the Developing World," *Foreign Affairs*, Vol. 75, No. 1, January/February 1996.

Logue, James, "Disasters, the Environment and Public Health: Improving Our Response," *American Journal of Public Health*, Vol. 86, No. 9, 1996.

Matthew, Richard, and George Shambaugh, "Sex, Drugs and Heavy Metal," *Security Dialogue*, Vol. 29, No. 2, 1998, p. 163.

McCarthy, James, Osvaldo Canziani, Neil Leary, David Dokken, and Kasey White, eds., *IPCC Third Assessment Report: Climate Change 2001—Impacts, Adaptation, and Vulnerability*, available at http://www.ipcc.ch/pub/reports.htm.

McLean, George, "The United Nations and the New Security Agenda," available at http://www.unac.org/canada/security/mclean.html.

McMichael, A., "Global Environmental Change and Human Population Health: A Conceptual and Scientific Challenge for Epidemiology," *International Journal of Epidemiology*, Vol. 22, 1993, pp. 1–8.

Medical Research Council (MRC) of South Africa, *The Impact of HIV/AIDS on Adult Mortality in South Africa*, available at http://www.mrc.ac.za.

Mills, Greg, "AIDS and the South African Military: Timeworn Cliché or Timebomb?" *HIV/AIDS: A Threat to the African Renaissance*, Konrad-Adenauer-Stiftung Occasional Papers, June 2000.

"More Thai Patients Progress to Full-Blown Disease," *Bangkok Post*, March 22, 2001.

Morse, Stephen S., "Controlling Infectious Diseases," Federation of American Scientists, available at http://www.fas.org/promed/papers/morse.htm, accessed July 11, 2001.

National Health Care Anti-Fraud Association, "Health-Care Fraud: A Serious and Costly Reality for All Americans," fact sheets, available at http://www.nhcaa.org/factsheet_impact.htm, accessed December 15, 2001.

National Institute of Allergy and Infectious Diseases (NIAID), "NIAID: Planning for the 21st Century," 2000, available at http://www. niaid.nih.gov/strategicplan2000/default.htm.

_____, "Infectious Diseases Research," available at http://www.niaid. nih.gov/eidr/mceid.htm, accessed July 5, 2001.

_____, "Antimicrobial Resistance," fact sheet, available at http://www.niaid.nih.gov/factsheets/antimicro.htm, accessed January 16, 2002.

National Intelligence Council (NIC), "The Global Infectious Disease Threat and Its Implications for the United States," NIE-99-17D, Washington, D.C., January 2000.

National Science and Technology Council, *Infectious Disease—A Global Health Threat*, report of the Committee on International Science, Engineering, and Technology, September 1995, available at http://www.state.gov/www/global/oes/health/task_force/wh thtreat.html, accessed June 28, 2001.

Naval Health Research Center, "DoD HIV/AIDS Prevention Program," available at http://www.nhrc.navy.mil/programs/life/ managementplan.html, accessed August 30, 2001.

"Needy Nation Struggles with Disaster, A," *Sydney Morning Herald*, September 19, 1998.

Nelson, Kenrad, "Thailand's HIV-Prevention Program Has Slowed the Epidemic, but AIDS-Related Opportunistic Infections Have Increased," Johns Hopkins School of Public Health, May 31, 2001, available at http://www.jhsph.edu/pubaffairs/press/thailands_ HIV.html.

Newburn, T., "Youth, Crime and Justice," in M. Maguire, R. Morgan, and R. Reiner, eds., *The Oxford Handbook of Criminology*, Oxford: Clarendon Press, 1997.

"Notice to Readers: Deferral of Routine Booster Doses of Tetanus and Diphtheria Toxoids for Adolescents and Adults," *MMWR*, Vol. 50, No. 20, May 25, 2001, pp. 418, 427.

O'Callaghan, M., "PNG-Positive," *Australian Magazine [Weekend Australian]*, November 13–14, 1999.

Ostroff, Stephen M., "The Epidemic Intelligence Service in the United States," *Eurosurveillance*, Vol. 6, No. 3, March 2001, pp. 34–36, available at http://www.ceses.org/eurosurveillance/V6n3/ En53-222.htm, accessed August 13, 2001.

"Out in the Open," *Newsweek*, December 4, 2000.

Pan, Philip P., "Scientists Issue Dire Prediction on Warming," *Washington Post*, January 23, 2001, p. A1.

Parry, Charles, *South African Community Epidemiology Network on Drug Use (SACENDU), January–June 1998 (Phase 4)*, available at http://www.mrc.ac.za.

Passel, J. S., and M. Fix, "US Immigration at the Beginning of the 21st Century," testimony before the Subcommittee on Immigration and Claims, U.S. House of Representatives, August 2, 2001 available at www.urban.org/TESTIMON/passel_fix_08-02-01.html, accessed on November 9, 2001.

Pianin, Eric, "U.N. Report Forecasts Crises Brought on by Global Warming," *Washington Post,* February 20, 2001, p. A6.

_____, "Two Studies Affirm Greenhouse Gases' Effects," *Washington Post,* April 13, 2001, p. A6.

_____, "Around Globe, Cities Have Growing Pains," *Washington Post,* June 11, 2001, p. A9.

Pirages, Dennis, "Microsecurity: Disease Organisms and Human Well-Being," *Washington Quarterly,* Vol. 18, No. 4, 1995.

"Polluted Environment Causing Worldwide Illness and Deaths," *Manila Times* (Philippines), May 24, 1998.

Pomerantsev, A. P., N. A. Staritsin, Y. V. Mockov, and L. I. Marinin, "Expression of Cereolysine AB Genes in Bacillus Anthracis Vaccine Strain Ensures Protection Against Experimental Hemolytic Anthrax Infection," *Vaccine,* Vol. 15, Nos. 17–18, December 1997, pp. 1846–1850.

"Preliminary FoodNet Data on the Incidence of Foodborne Illnesses—Selected Sites, United States, 2000," *MMWR,* Vol. 50, No. 13, April 6, 2001, pp. 241–246, available at http://www.cdc.gov/mmwr/preview/mmwrhtml/mm5013a1.htm accessed June 21, 2002.

Purver, Ron, "Chemical, Biological, Radiological and Nuclear (CBRN) Terrorism," Perspectives Report 2000/02, Ottawa: CSIS, December 18, 1999.

_____, "Chemical and Biological Terrorism: A New Threat to Public Safety?" *Conflict Studies,* Vol. 295, 1996.

Quinn, Thomas, "The AIDS Epidemic: Demographic Aspects, Population Biology and Virus Evolution," in Richard Krause, ed., *Emerging Infections,* New York: Academic Press, 1998, p. 331.

_____, "Population Migration and the Spread of Types I and 2 Human Immunodeficiency Viruses," in Bernard Roizman, ed.,

Infectious Diseases in an Age of Change, Washington, D.C.: National Academy Press, 1995, p. 81.

"Raining Misery: Millions Marooned in Bangladesh," *Sydney Morning Herald,* September 19, 1998.

Reingold, Arthur, "Outbreak Investigations—A Perspective," *Emerging Infectious Diseases,* Vol. 4, No. 1, January–March 1998, available at http://www.cdc.gov/ncidod/EID/vol4no1/reingold.htm.

"Rise of the Megacity," *The Australian,* April 24, 1997.

Roizman, Bernard, ed., *Infectious Diseases in an Age of Change,* Washington, D.C.: National Academy Press, 1995.

Rosenau, James, *Turbulence in World Politics: A Theory of Change and Continuity,* Princeton, N.J.: Princeton University Press, 1990.

Rosenthal, Elisabeth, "In Rural China, a Steep Price for Poverty: Dying of AIDS," *New York Times,* October 28, 2000, p. A1.

_____, "With Ignorance as the Fuel, AIDS Speeds Across China," *New York Times,* December 30, 2001, p. A1.

Roush, Sandra, Guthrie Birkhead, Denise Koo, Angela Cobb, and David Fleming, "Mandatory Reporting of Diseases and Conditions by Health Care Professionals and Laboratories," *JAMA,* Vol. 282, No. 2, July 14, 1999.

"S. African Says AIDS Not Biggest Killer," *Washington Post,* August 7, 2001.

Schmid, Ray, "Post Office Turns to Congress for Financial Help," Associated Press, November 8, 2001, available at http://sns.kcpq.com/sns-anthrax-mail.story.

Schoch-Spana, M., "Hospitals Buckle During Normal Flu Season: Implications for Bioterrorism Response," *Biodefense Quarterly,* Vol. 1, No. 4, March 2000, available at http://www.hopkins-biodefense.org/pages/news/quarter1_4.html, accessed December 15, 2001.

Schönteich, Martin, "AIDS and Age: SA's Crime Time Bomb?" *AIDS Analysis Africa,* Vol. 10, No. 2, 1999. p. 1.

____, "Age and AIDS: A Lethal Mix for South Africa's Crime Rate," *HIV/AIDS: A Threat to the African Renaissance?* Konrad-Adenauer-Stiftung Occasional Papers, June 2000.

____, "The Impact of HIV/AIDS on South Africa's Internal Security," paper delivered at the First Annual Conference of the South African Association of Public Administration and Management, Pretoria, November 23, 2000.

Schwartz, B., D. Bell, and J. M. Hughes, "Preventing the Emergence of Antimicrobial Resistance: A Call for Action by Clinicians, Public Health Officials, and Patients," *JAMA*, Vol. 278, No. 11, September 17, 1997, pp. 901–904.

Shaw, Martin, *Global Society and International Relations*, Cambridge, Mass.: Polity Press, 1994.

"Sheep Smuggled from Yemen Responsible for Jizan Outbreak," *Arab News*, September 24, 2000.

Shell, Robert, "Halfway to the Holocaust: The Economic, Demographic and Social Implications of the AIDS Pandemic to the Year 2010 in the Southern African Region," in *HIV/AIDS: A Threat to the African Renaissance?* Konrad-Adenauer-Stiftung Occasional Papers, June 2000.

"60% of [South African] Army May Be HIV Positive," *Mail and Guardian* (South Africa), March 31, 2000.

Skeel, Michael R., "Toward a National Laboratory System for Public Health," *Emerging Infectious Diseases*, Vol. 7, No. 3, Supplement, June 2001, p. 531.

Smith, Joseph, "The Threat of New Infectious Diseases," *Journal of the Royal Society of Medicine*, Vol. 86, 1993.

Smith, T. L., M. L. Pearson, K. R. Wilcox, C. Cruz, M. V. Lancaster, and B. Robinson-Dunn, "Emergence of Vancomycin Resistance in *Staphylococcus aureus*," *New England Journal of Medicine*, Vol. 340, 1999, pp. 493–501.

Smithson, Amy E., and Leslie-Anne Levy, *Ataxia: The Chemical and Biological Terrorism Threat and the U.S. Response*, Stimson Center

Report No. 35, available at www.stimson.org/cbw/pubs.cfm? ID=12, p. 256.

Snow, Donald, *National Security: Enduring Problems in a Changing Defense Environment*, New York: St. Martin's Press, 1991.

Snyder, James W., and William Check, *Bioterrorism Threats to Our Future: The Role of the Clinical Microbiology Laboratory in Detection, Identification and Confirmation of Biological Agents*, Washington, D.C.: American Academy of Microbiology, 2001, p. 8.

"South Africa Must Dispense AIDS Drug to Pregnant Women," *New York Times*, December 14, 2001.

South African Health Review, 2000, available at http://www.hst. org.za/sahr/2000.

"Spectre Stalking the Sub-Sahara, The," *The Economist*, December 2, 2000.

Speed, Steyn, "ANC Pamphlet on World AIDS Day," available at http://lists.sn.apc.org/pipermail/election2000/20001201/000082. html.

Suhkre, Astri, "Human Security and the Interest of States," *Security Dialogue*, Vol. 30, No. 3, 1999, p. 269.

Teklehaimanot, A., "Travel Report to Ethiopia," unpublished WHO report, 1991.

"Ten Great Public Health Achievements, 1900–1999," *MMWR*, available at http://www.cdc.gov/od/nvpo/arttop10.htm, accessed October 15, 2001.

"Terrorism and the Warfare of the Weak," *The Guardian* (UK), October 27, 1993.

"Terrorism Is Not the Only Scourge," *The Economist*, December 22, 2001.

"Thai Army Winning AIDS Battle," *Far Eastern Economic Review*, May 5, 1998.

Thakur, Ramesh, "From National to Human Security," in Stuart Harris and Andrew Mack, eds., *Asia-Pacific Security: The Economics-Politics Nexus,* Sydney: Allen and Unwin, 1997.

"They Survived Mitch—To Live in Misery," *Sunday Times* (Singapore), November 15, 1998.

Thompson, Tommy G., Secretary, HHS, testimony before the Subcommittee on Commerce, Justice, State, and Judiciary, Committee on Appropriations, U.S. Senate, May 9, 2001, available at http:// www.os.dhhs.gov/progorg/asl/testify/t010509.html, accessed September 3, 2001.

Thomson American Healthcare Consultants, "Guidelines for Prevention and Control of Pandemic Influenza in Healthcare Institutions," March 23, 2000, available at http://www.ahcpub.com/ ahc_root_html/hot/breakingnews/flu03232000.html, accessed March 16, 2002.

Tow, William, "Linkages Between Traditional Security and Human Security," in William Tow, Ramesh Thakur, and In-Taek Hyun, eds., *Asia's Emerging Regional Order: Reconciling Traditional and Human Security,* Tokyo: United Nations University Press, 2000.

Tucker, Jonathan B., "National Health and Medical Services Response to Incidents of Chemical and Biological Terrorism," *JAMA,* Vol. 278, No. 5, 1997, pp. 362–368, available at http://www. lsic.ucla.edu/classes/mimg/spring01/micro12/Website/JAMAarti cles/response.html, accessed July 5, 2001.

United Nations, "UN Anti-Aids Effort Enlists Coca-Cola to Curb Spread of Epidemic in Africa," June 21, 2000, available at http:// allafrica.com/stories/200106210333.html.

UNAIDS, *The Status and Trends of the Global HIV/AIDS Pandemic,* Geneva: UNAIDS Publication, July 1996.

_____, *HIV/AIDS: The Global Epidemic,* Geneva: UNAIDS Publication, December 1996.

_____, "AIDS Hits Asia Hard," December 1997, available at http:// www.thalidomide.org/FfdN/Asien/asia.html.

_____, *AIDS Epidemic Update—December 2001*, available at http://www.unaids.org/publications/index.html.

UNAIDS/WHO Working Group on Global HIV/AIDS and STD Surveillance, "Epidemiological Fact Sheet on HIV/AIDS and Sexually Transmitted Diseases—South Africa" (including updates), available at http://www.who.ch/emc/diseases/hiv.

"Update: Investigation of Bioterrorism-Related Anthrax and Interim Guidelines for Exposure Management and Antimicrobial Therapy, October 2001," *MMWR*, Vol. 50, No. 42, October 26, 2001, pp. 910–919, available at http://www.cdc.gov/mmwr/preview/mmwr html/mm5042a1.htm, accessed June 22, 2002.

U.S. Agency for International Development (USAID), "Reducing the Threat of Infectious Diseases of Major Public Health Importance: USAID's Initiative to Prevent and Control Infectious Diseases," March 1998, p. 3, available at www.usaid.gov/pop_health/pdf/idfstrategy.pdf.

_____, "USAID: Leading the Global Fight Against HIV/AIDS," available at http://www.usaid.gov/press/releases/2001/fs010420_4. html, accessed August 13, 2001.

U.S. Army Medical Research and Materiel Command, "RAD 1—Military Infectious Disease Research Program," available at http://mrmc-www.army.mil/, accessed October 15, 2001.

U.S. Army Technical Escort Unit, Web page, available at http://teu.sbccom.army.mil/index.htm, accessed September 6, 2001.

U.S. Department of Agriculture (USDA)/FSIS, "Protecting the Public from Foodborne Illness: The Food Safety Inspection Service," April 2001, available at http://www.fsis.usda.gov/oa/background/fsisgeneral.htm, accessed July 24, 2001.

U.S. Department of Health and Human Services (HHS), "Medical Response in Emergencies: HHS Role," fact sheet, January 25, 2001, available at http://www.os.dhhs.gov/news/press/2001pres/01fs emergencyresponse.html, accessed July 6, 2001.

_____, "Antimicrobial Resistance: The Public Health Response," fact sheet, available at http://www.hhs.gov/news/press/2001pres/01 fsdrugresistance.html, accessed June 28, 2001.

_____, Office of Emergency Preparedness, "NDMS: Catastrophic Care for the Nation," available at http://ndms.dhhs.gov/NDMS/ndms.html, accessed July 2, 2001.

_____, "Office of Emergency Preparedness," available at http://www. oep.dhhs.gov/, accessed July 6, 2001.

_____, "FY 2002 President's Budget for HHS," p. 33, available at http://www.hhs.gov/budget/pdf/h.PDF, accessed August 30, 2001.

U.S. Department of State, "United States Strategy on HIV/AIDS," publication no. 10296 (July 1995), available at http://dosfan.lib. uic.edu/ERC/environment/releases/9507.html, p. 30.

_____, "Fact Sheet on South Africa," available at http://www.state. gov/r/pa/bgn/index.

U.S. Senate, "Bioterrorism: Public Health and Medical Preparedness," statement by Janet Heinrich, October 9, 2001, before the Senate Subcommittee on Public Health, GAO-02-141T,

_____, testimony of Tracy Mehan, Assistant Administrator for Water, U.S. Environmental Protection Agency, before the Committee on Environment and Public Works, Subcommittee on Fisheries, Wildlife, and Water, October 31, 2001, available at http://www.win-water.org/win_legislative/win_testimony/103101mehan.html, accessed November 30, 2001).

Venter, Al, "Biological Warfare: The Poor Man's Atomic Bomb," *Jane's Intelligence Review*, March 1999.

Vogt, Donna U., "CRS Issue Brief for Congress: Food Safety Issues in the 106th Congress," February 12, 1999, available at http://www.csa.com/hottopics/ern/99jul/ag-38.html, accessed December 15, 2001.

Wedding and Event Videographers Association (WEVA),"US Post Office Acquires Irradiation Technology," October 28, 2001, available at http://www.weva.com/cgi-bin/newsreader.pl?storyid=255&type=I.

Weinstein, Robert, "Nosocomial Infection Update," *Emerging Infectious Diseases,* Vol. 4, No. 3, 1998, available at http://www.cdc.gov/ncidod/eid/vol4no3/weinstein.htm, accessed December 7, 2000.

"White House Sets Out Blueprint for Homeland Security," *Financial Times,* June 19, 2002.

White House, The, Office of Science and Technology Policy, "Addressing the Threat of Emerging Infectious Diseases," PDD/NSTC-7, June 12, 1996, available at http://www.state.gov/www/global/oes/health/task_force/whthtreat.html, accessed June 28, 2001.

Whiteside, Alan, "HIV/AIDS Implications for Poverty Reduction," *United Nations Development Programme Policy Paper,* 2000, pp. 5–10.

_____, and David FitzSimons, "The AIDS Epidemic: Economic, Political and Security Implications," *Conflict Studies,* Vol. 251, 1992.

_____, and Clem Sunter, *AIDS: The Challenge for South Africa,* Cape Town: Human and Rousseau Tafelberg, 2000.

"WIIO Cites Air Travel Risk," Associated Press (AP), December 18, 1998.

Wills, Christopher, *Plagues: Their Origin, History and Future,* London: Flamingo Books, 1997.

"Wonder Drugs at Risk," *Washington Post,* April 19, 2001, p. A18.

Woolsey, James, quoted in John Ciccarelli, "Preface: Instruments of Darkness—Crime and Australian National Security," in John Ciccarelli, ed., *Transnational Crime: A New Security Threat?* Canberra: Australian Defence Studies Centre, 1996, p. xi.

World Bank, "Macroeconomics and Health: Investing in Health for Economic Development," report of the World Bank Commission on Macroeconomics and Health, December 2001, available at http://www.cmhealth.org/index.html.

World Bank Group, "India's National AIDS Control Program," September 1999, available at http://www.worldbank.org/aids.

World Health Organization (WHO), "Report on Infectious Diseases: Removing Obstacles to Healthy Development," available at http://www.who.org/infectious-disease-report/pages/textonly.html, pp. 1–2.

_____, *Removing Obstacles to Healthy Development: WHO Report on Infectious Diseases*, 1999, available at http://www.who.org/home/reports.html, accessed January 15, 1999.

_____, *Overcoming Antimicrobial Resistance*, 2000, available at www.who.int/infectious-disease-report/.

Yach, Derek, "The Globalization of Public Health I: Threats and Opportunities," *American Journal of Public Health,* Vol. 88, No. 5. 1998.

"Young Bear the Brunt as AIDS Spreads Through the World on a Biblical Scale," *The Independent*, November 25, 1998.

"Young, Gifted and Dead," *Sunday Times* (South Africa), July 9, 2000.